Writing Blackgirls' and Women's Health Science

Writing Blackgirls' and Women's Health Science

Implications for Research and Praxis

Edited by
Jameta Nicole Barlow

LEXINGTON BOOKS
Lanham • Boulder • New York • London

Published by Lexington Books
An imprint of The Rowman & Littlefield Publishing Group, Inc.
4501 Forbes Boulevard, Suite 200, Lanham, Maryland 20706
www.rowman.com

86-90 Paul Street, London EC2A 4NE

British Library Cataloguing in Publication Information Available

Library of Congress Cataloging-in-Publication Data

Names: Barlow, Jameta Nicole, editor.
Title: Writing Black girls' and women's health science : implications for research and praxis / edited by Jameta Nicole Barlow.
Description: Lanham : Lexington Books, [2024] | Includes bibliographical references and index.
Identifiers: LCCN 2023042868 (print) | LCCN 2023042869 (ebook) | ISBN 9781666911749 (cloth) | ISBN 9781666911756 (ebook)
Subjects: LCSH: African American women—Medical care—Research. | African American girls—Medical care—Research. | African American women—Health and hygiene—Research. | African American girls—Health and hygiene—Research.
Classification: LCC RA564.86 .W75 2024 (print) | LCC RA564.86 (ebook) | DDC 362.1089/96073—dc23/eng/20231011
LC record available at https://lccn.loc.gov/2023042868
LC ebook record available at https://lccn.loc.gov/2023042869

This book is dedicated to all the Blackgirls and women who were failed and ignored by the healthcare system . . . and erased from the scientific process. A special dedication to Black women who transitioned too soon, including my college roommate, friend, and sister by choice Tamika W. McDowell-Randolph. We offer a new way of doing Blackgirls' and women's health, so no more Black women die prematurely.

Contents

List of Figures and Tables ix

1 Philosophies of Blackgirls' and Women's Health Science 1
Jameta Nicole Barlow

2 Out of Racism, The Scholar 15
Linda Goler Blount

3 BlackGirl Wellness 31
LeConté J. Dill

4 The Utility of Love for Black Women's Health 43
Breya Johnson

5 The Stories We Hold: Health Implications of Embodied Narratives of Black Women and Girls from the Ivory Tower 57
Chinyere Okafor

6 Welcome to the Kitchen Table: Where Stories and Images Center the Lived Experiences of Black Women and Their Bodies 77
Y. Falami Devoe

7 Lifting as I Climb, Resting When I Need To 95
Shawn Arango Ricks

8 "If You Can't Relate to Me, How Can You Treat Me?": Centering Black Girls' Voices in Culturally Responsive Health Praxis 109
Maryam M. Jernigan-Noesi

9 Using the Guided Hair Autobiography for Black Women and Girls as a Health Assessment 123
Afiya Mbilishaka

10 Breaking the Concrete Ceiling: Shifting and Stress Among Black Women in the Workplace 139
Danielle Dickens

11 Eluding the White Gaze: Sex Education for Black Girls by Black Women 147
Sara C. Flowers

12 Black Women Stay Fighting Structural Racism: Other-mothering as Community Praxis 167
Maranda Ward

13 Our WISH for Black Girls' and Women's Health: Women, Intersectionality, Science and Health (WISH) Writing Lab 185
Breya Johnson, Toni Junious, Martha Kakooza, Carlysha Isaac, Juliette Garofolo, Danielle Whyte, Madelyn Stalter

14 The Afterword: Reimagining Black Health 201
Melicia C. Whitt-Glover, Olivia Affuso, Tambra Raye Stevenson, Jameta Nicole Barlow, Shiriki K. Kumanyika (On Behalf of the Council on Black Health)

Index 221

About the Editor 233

About the Contributors 235

List of Figures and Tables

FIGURES

Figure 1.1 Black Girls' and Women's Health Philosophy of Science 3
Figure 11.1 Multidimensional Power: An Intersectional Sexuality Education Model 154

TABLE

Table 8.1 Black Girls' Coping Strategies 115

Chapter 1

Philosophies of Blackgirls' and Women's Health Science

Jameta Nicole Barlow

Language is the expression of thought and action. When language is read or written, it has the ability to open a window to imagination, communication, history, and perspective. The written word is a very powerful weapon—it can inspire and persuade. For example, while there are archeological reports suggesting 5% of enslaved individuals learned how to read before the American Revolution (Bly, 2021), the act of reading and writing was considered illegal in all U.S. slave states except for Maryland, Kentucky, and Tennessee (Smithsonian, 2022). The people in power knew that the people not in power would organize and fight for their freedom through shared language and agency. This is why enslaved Africans from similar nations, language, and culture were intentionally separated during the TransAtlantic Slave Trade. This also explains why it was forbidden for groups of enslaved Black people to gather outside of working, why names were changed, why traditional religions and spiritual practices were forbidden, and why Christianity was only allowed. And, why they exerted control over the enslaved individuals' bodily autonomy and agency, specifically language.

Liberation is inextricably linked to reading and writing. Many of the slave states passed laws against teaching enslaved individuals to read and write after the 1831 Nat Turner Rebellion, where an enslaved Virginian and man of faith named Nat Turner taught himself to read and write and debunked common thought that enslaved individuals were happy and docile by organizing the Rebellion also known as the Southampton Insurrection in August 1831, resulting in the killings of 51 white Virginians (Coleman, 2021). His reading, writing, visions, and faith had to result in liberation. The institution of slavery stripped Black people of our humanity—where any expression of culture (e.g., speaking native languages, names, religion, etc.) could result in death. But the ideologies and systems that created and upheld the peculiar institution of slavery, especially in the Americas and as a result of the TransAtlantic Slave Trade, set the standard for scientific inquiry. This book contributes to the burgeoning literature working toward Black women–informed and engaged philosophies of Black girls' and women's health sciences.

WORDS ARE POWERFUL

The name of this book is very intentional: *Writing Black Girls' and Women's Health Science: Implications for Research and Praxis.* May this book inspire future writers, scholars, activists, and researchers focused on the doing of Black girls' and women's health (BGWH). The objective is to persuade them to consider their philosophy of science—their ways of knowing—our ways of knowing—specifically their ontologies (what is knowledge) and epistemologies (how we come to know and do knowledge)—in their work on BGWH. And, perhaps consider ancestral and spiritual knowledges' influence on BGWH as well (Some, 1997). Negotiating these ways of knowing prior to moving forward with their methodologies may serve as a decolonized approach to science and health, as it requires one to interrogate their knowledge on the subject of inquiry, and consider how that knowledge was developed, prior to deciding how to explore the subject of inquiry. How we write and what we write is directly related to who we are, as well as our ontologies and epistemologies.

MY PHILOSOPHY OF SCIENCE

My philosophy of science (figure 1.1), framed by Black Feminism, Womanism, the Southern Black Feminisms Health Framework (Barlow & Smith, 2019) and the Black Feminist and Womanist (BFW) Analytical Path to Health Equity (Barlow & Johnson, 2021) was the impetus for the 2018 special issue on Black women's health calling for interdisciplinary and transdisciplinary approaches to BGWH; organizing the 2018 Re-Imagining Black Girls' and Women's Health Symposium and Workshop at Towson University (#ReclaimingBGWH); development of a writing course on Black girls' and women's health; a Black Girls' and Women's Health Research and Praxis Collaborative; several workshops and conference presentations on public health and psychology; women's studies conferences and conventions; and recognizing the need for this book.

Black women be knowing.

And it is that knowledge that has created systems, institutions, and transformed lives. This country is built upon Black women's wombs. And, the path forward is not only by listening to Black women (Barlow, 2021), but

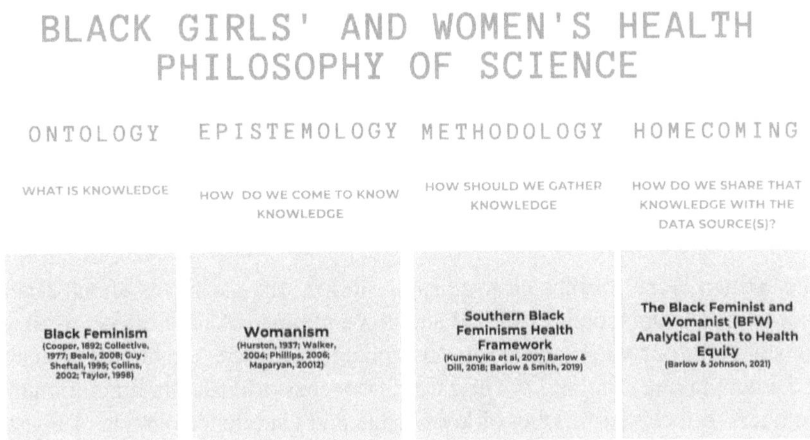

Figure 1.1 Black Girls' and Women's Health Philosophy of Science. *Source*: Created by author.

also by unapologetically recognizing that we have another knowledge system that has sustained us and framed our lived experiences, despite structural oppressions. This knowledge system comes from Black women, is curated by Black women, and should be returned to Black women to ensure consistency with our knowledge systems. And while we know we cannot change the structures using the tools that designed the structure (Lorde, 1984), we know that we have our own structures that have sustained us, provided for us, and continue to offer a balm amidst the storm and chaos that can be the Blackgirl lived experience. It is imperative that we use Blackgirl knowledge systems to transform Blackgirl lives and to share with other Blackgirls. This work is not just for me. It is for all the generations that are to come after me, but especially honoring those Blackgirls who have paved the way and prayed for books just like this.

We are all too familiar with the knowledge handed down mother to daughter and back to mother and daughter, as expressed by Michelle T. Berger's (2021) cheers for the organizers of healing spaces and research collaboratives that like us, understand, we know what we need: for us, by us. This is why our cover, wonderfully created by the Washington, DC Takoma neighborhood artist, Tarika Art, hopefully represents the care with which we hand down information for generations forward. We subvert notions of whiteness, patriarchy, and capitalism as the gold standard for health behaviors, frameworks, theories, and methodologies when we have epistemologists such as granny midwives, birthworkers, community healers, church women, hair stylists, conjurers, herbalists, and naturopaths with ways of knowing that have carried us over generations. The SARS-COV2/COVID19 pandemic ignited many to revisit these ancestral epistemologies and engage in related methodologies, connecting with the earth and re-engaging communities around farming, gardening, yoga, diet, and herbal remedies. We return to our roots because they sustain us.

THE WRITTEN PATH

The written word enables us to tell our stories, our narratives about experiences and accounts, both historical and contemporary. And, it allows us to tell the stories in our way, situated in positionality. Howard University professor and ardent public scholar, Dr. Greg Carr, convenes office hours for community members to receive a sharing of knowledge and experience outside of his students. In December 2021 on the popular Black-owned social media hub "Knubia," Dr. Carr explained that "The language contains the key to the culture." This is why the languages of enslaved African people were forbidden from being spoken and speakers of different languages were intentionally mixed. We are currently relearning, or rather reacquainting ourselves with knowledges, rooted in African ways of knowing. And, according to Dr. Carr, "You can't fix this culture—it's in the language." Thus, this book does not seek to fix the culture of scientific inquiry about BGWH. Instead, we will use the colonizing language in our own way—remixing academic jargon with our communities' vernacular—to make our knowledges accessible and alive in our communities. This means we may or may not wax poetic about how the ways of knowing (and doing), such as those archived in the *Southern Medical Journal,* were rooted in what our beloved bell hooks called "imperialist-white-supremacist-capitalist-patriarchy" (hooks, 2005), the ideology framing settler colonialism (Dunbar, 2014). This way of knowing and doing work about and on Black girls and women have contributed to the current state of BGWH. Much of what we know about BGWH prior to the 1900s was based on diaries, notes, journals, and publications through the lens of white men. Whenever Black women exhibit agency, and share knowledge with one another, we become a threat to the health establishment (e.g., *Sheppard Towner Act of 1921* and its effect on the amelioration of granny midwives). The liberation of Black people, Black women, and Black families was a threat to the status of white slave owners. In spite of enslavement, Black women found ways to share information when the laws and the rules did not allow them to be vocal or viewed as experts.

> To abort unwanted pregnancies, slave women sometimes used the cotton plant, the staple crop of the South. The root of the cotton plant could be made into a tea or chewed.45 By terminating a pregnancy that would have resulted in an

> additional worker for the slave owner, and by utilizing the plant that provided him income, the female slave was exercising some control over her body and her enslaved situation. (Sullivan, 2010; Schwartz, 2010)

This book moves across the personal narrative, academic jargon, and scholar activism, resulting in a bidirectional relationship of theory and praxis for our communities. And, yes, for us.

WE ARE THE INTERVENTION

As former Blackgirls, now Black women, our mere presence in professional spaces is often an unintentional intervention. However, this book is intentional. We are embracing and using language to engage Black women's intellectual thought, because ultimately, as history has repeatedly demonstrated, Black women's ways, words, and wonders will save ourselves. We, Black folx, have always been content creators—in music, from work songs while enslaved, to the evolution of Black music—spirituals, blues, jazz, rhythm and blues, hip hop, and neo-soul to the popular social media TikTok dances. Black communities create, and too often our art, our knowledge, and our spirit, rooted in African and ancestral knowing, are stolen, repackaged, and fed to us as popular music or the latest craze. The same has happened in BGWH. Granny midwives and what we would call birthworkers today were the primary catchers of babies (Sullivan, 2010) during U.S. slavery; yet, midwives became marginalized in the South in the 1900s. Today, doulas and birthworkers are touted as the cure to addressing adverse maternal health outcomes. We know what we need and must inspire and persuade. We must build our interventions, policies, and work around Black intellectual thought, Black women's ways of knowing, and in the name of science and medicine.

There is a developing canon of research on the lived experiences of Black girls and women, which we know are the major determinants of health for BGWH. We build upon the continuing legacies of the Black Women's Health Imperative birthed by Byllye Avery and so many other Black women comrades, currently under the leadership of Linda Goler Blount, for whom we are honored by her foreword of this edited collection. We support the data collection and analysis the Boston Black Women's Health Study has provided to the field for decades. We engage in effective allyship (Preston, 2018), and sometimes co-conspiratorship with femmes and trans women of color, both populations that experience some of the highest levels of adverse health outcomes and are often ignored and erased from the data. We acknowledge the works of Moya Bailey and Whitney Peoples (2017) in their articulation of a Black feminist health sciences study that bridges health sciences with public thought. We are stimulated by Stephanie Evans' historical and archival work that chronicles Black women's words, lives, and strategies for wellness, even uncovering a now widely shared picture of Rosa Parks practicing yoga (2019). We unapologetically approach science engaging in Black Feminisms, as articulated by Venus Evans-Winters (2010). There are so many scholars who already interrogate philosophies and reimagine Black futures and realities that are engaging in spaces often marginalized within our communities. From gender interrogations (Bey, 2019) to Black women's culture and its entanglements with U.S. imperialism (Edwards, 2021) to Black aesthetics as resistance (Jones, 2020) and the representation of women's lives (King, 2019), explicating the language of Black feminist legal theory (Randolph, 2017), especially with respect to Black reproductive justice, Black mysticisms (Warren, 2017) to Diasporic dreaming (Williams, 2018). There is a place for all of us and our approaches to this work that we have been called to do in the name of BGWH.

We do not describe health issues affecting BGWH, using a deficit approach and then offer solutions using a westernized approach. Instead, we offer Black women informed, lived, and engaged philosophies to reframe the health narrative and praxis of Black girls' and women's health. As a result, we don't have to talk about the historical exclusion of Black communities. Instead, we offer language that centers the lived experiences of Black girls and women. This book introduces a Blackgirls' and women's health (BGWH) philosophy of science, framework, and guide for writing about Blackgirls' and women's health. Our goal is to transform how Blackgirls' and women's health science is studied, taught, and conducted in research, praxis, and clinical spaces. This book is for three audiences

1. the average community member seeking to create change in their neighborhood and looking for narratives of change that validate what they already know must be done in order to center Black women and healing;
2. the practitioner, scholar, researcher, organizer also seeking validation and confirmation for what they already know needs to be done in their area of focus; and,
3. everyone, because we need new ways of knowing and being—an expansion of what BGWH science looks like.

Focus of the Work

In a 1975 keynote address at Portland State University, Toni Morrison said, "The function, the very serious function of racism is distraction. It keeps you from doing your work. It keeps you explaining, over and over again, your reason for being. Somebody says you have no language and you spend twenty years proving that you do. Somebody says your head isn't shaped properly so you have scientists working on the fact that it is. Somebody says you have no art, so you dredge that up. Somebody says you have no kingdoms, so you dredge that up. None of this is necessary. There will always be one more thing" (Morrison et al., 1975; Barajas, 2019). We are not in a deficit of literature describing the status and explaining the health outcomes disproportionately affecting BGWH. This descriptive and explanatory work is important, foundational, and necessary to the BGWH canon. Yet, this book is not that work. We are not distracted.

In this edited collection of BGWH philosophies, we do less descriptive and explanatory writing and more declarative, community, and action-based writing about BGWH. We may mention the institutions that created our current health status, but we center Black women's knowledge and philosophies of science to achieve optimal health. Readers will turn each page of this book, transformed by each word, each philosophy, or chapter, that is shared about BGWH. In these pages, we will not justify our framing, use of critical race theory, intersectionality, and the Combahee River Collective's notion of identity politics. The work we are doing here is not to justify our philosophy, but simply stating that we will frame, write, think, and organize for our healing and well-being. Our beloved bell hooks repeatedly reminded us our walk in this world is theory and that way of knowing and doing is useful, fruitful, and enough. Simply put, we are enough.

We acknowledge the Native/Indigenous intellectual thought of decolonizing methodologies and the need to disrupt settler colonialism

> "Nation. race. and class converged in land" Everything in US history is about the land—who oversaw and cultivated it, fished its waters, maintained its wildlife, who invaded and stole it; how it became a commodity ("real estate") broken into pieces to be bought and sold on the market . . . . The history of the United States is a history of settler colonialism—the founding of a state based on the ideology of white supremacy, the widespread practice of African slavery, and a policy of genocide and land theft. (Dunbar-Ortiz, 2014)

This cues us to uncover new languages and terms to design a BGWH science for ourselves.

Standing on the narratives and words of so many ways of knowing for BGWH, we offer a Black girls' and women's health science philosophy from A to Z—Anna Julia Hayward Cooper to Zora Neale Hurston—traipsing across the intellectual terrain of Black Feminists and Womanists who have shaped contemporary thought on BGWH in the most culturally and structurally competent fashion that not only invokes the ancestors who imagined better times, but also Black midwives, birthworkers, conjurers of dreams and realities, and healers who still maintain the health of Black communities.

(RE)-CLAIMING BLACK GIRLS' AND WOMEN'S HEALTH (#RECLAIMINGBGWH)

There is a movement to re-claim BGWH, despite the acknowledgment that the Black body is in constant conflict with the state (criminal justice, legislative) and at home (interpersonal and sexual violence, community violence). It is hard to reclaim something you may not have felt like you owned.

We Claim Ourselves: Ontologies

The liberation of American Black women did not start in the 1960s. Although not formally recognized until the second wave of the feminist movement, Black Feminism has manifested itself in works and efforts of social activists in the African American community such as Ida B. Wells Barnett, Mary McLeod Bethune, Anna Julia Cooper, Frances E.W. Harper, Maria Stewart, Mary Church Terrell, and Sojourner Truth. Much of the legacy of Black feminism is its efforts to solidify a Black Feminist Consciousness that seeks transformative change in the daily lives of Black women, their families, and communities. Black Feminism is entrenched in what Taylor describes as "…the glorious tradition of black female activists' trenchant commitment to empowering themselves to create a humanistic community" (Taylor, 1998).

Black Feminism resists oppression, and subverts marginalizing structures and the practices and ideas that justify it. It aims to empower Black women within the context of social justice sustained by intersecting oppressions. Foremother to both the feminist and Black Feminist canon, Raleigh, North Carolina native, Dr. Anna Julia Haywood Cooper's (b. Raleigh, NC August 10, 1858–February 27, 1964) lifetime efforts were rooted in transformational community-based action-oriented work, engaging upon principles of consciousness-raising, self-determination, agency, activism, and social change. Considered an original author of the Black Feminist intellectual tradition, Dr. Cooper boldly pronounced in 1938:

> The Colored woman today occupies, one may say, a unique position in this
>
> country. . . . She is confronted by both a woman question and a race problem, and is as yet
>
> an unknown or an unacknowledged factor in both[vii].

Although any one woman's experience is not a monolithic experience for all Black women, there are core themes that unite Black women and serve as a bridge between practice and thought. The narrative of Black women operates as a heterogeneous collective that is neither performative nor descriptive. It has the potential to ignite empathy and connect cultures through the lenses of multiple oppressions. These "self-defined standpoints" can also stimulate resistance. This was the essential message of the pioneering Black women at the 1978 Combahee Feminist Collective[viii]: to define, outline, advocate, and name their work as part of a political movement based upon the intersection of their race and gender, among other identities and structural oppressions. Dr. Patricia Hill Collins posited that there is a "connection between experience and consciousness that shapes the everyday lives of individual African American women" (2002; 1998) that often pervades the works of Black women activists and scholars. She considered this disconnect between experience and consciousness, which requires self-reflexivity; experience and ideas; practice and thought; where "intellectuals" and the ability to change in response to the time is critical not only to a grassroots effort, but particularly relevant for reigniting an intergenerational, social change agenda among Black women living in a social structure that encourages unhealthy living and care for others; delimiting self-care practices for Black women. Womanism offers such a methodology for connecting experience and Black Feminist consciousness around social change such as health disparities among Black women.

Alternatively, self-identifying as a Black woman is not a requirement in Black Feminist Ontologies. Dr. Beverly Guy-Sheftall contends Black feminisms are not exclusive to femaleness[x]. Rather, men can be Black feminists because the struggle for equality for Black girls and women is centralized around both experiences and ideas. In fact, Black Feminist Ontology as a point of analysis is not limited by race, sex, gender, sexuality, class, ability, or any other identity, though race and gender are more often foregrounded. Similarly, although feminism is for everybody, as advocated by bell hooks (2000), Black Feminism is for everybody. When the marginalized are centered, everyone benefits. In public health, we are often motivated to address the health needs of individuals and populations most at risk for a condition or disease. When Black Feminism is for everybody, as a tool of policy analysis, program development, and theoretical framework, the needs of the most marginalized groups in the United States can be addressed. This action centers the experience of Black women and elevates the collective gaze of all, such that, if Black girls and women aren't succeeding in a specific life domain (e.g., health, education, employment, etc.), then social structures should be examined by those administering these services to ensure optimal health.

Despite the existing seminal work in Black Feminist Studies, there still remains a narrow pathway of literature tapping into the feminist concerns of Black girls and women at all socio-economic levels and that takes into account the role of intersectionality in segmenting health attitudes, behaviors, and actions. Further, Black girls cannot succeed in educational contexts if they are not healthy. There is an opportunity for Black Feminist principles and practices to engage with Womanist methodologies and modalities to address BGWH.

Layli Maparyan suggests there are foundational methods that extend this and Womanism is a theoretical paradigm into one that is both healing and transformative as a methodology or modality[xviii]. These eight foundational methods seek to transform the complex multiple dimensions of health affecting the daily lives of women of color and include: self-care healing and wellness practices; harmonizing and coordinating; dialogue and the power of the word; arbitration and mediation; spiritual activities; hospitality; mutual aid and self-help; and motherhood. Womanist epistemologies and modalities can work in concert with Black Feminist ontologies to improve the health of Black women.

What is necessary is an evidence-base of literature that extends the current discourse in theorizing Black Feminisms (James, 2000) and Womanism, and their utility for transformational change in the lives of Black girls and women. Writing BGWH science requires heeding Toni Morrison's advice, in spite of the structural barriers toward progress. The following ontological leanings are offered as principles upon which this book can be read, entrenched in Black Feminism, Black Feminist and Womanist Thought, and Black Feminist Consciousness: power of the personal narrative; quest for intersectional equality balance grounded in gendered and racialized consciousness; individual and collective agency as a political movement; and generational wealth of knowledge and pursuit.

ABOUT THIS EDITED COLLECTION

Through time and place, thought and praxis, joy and healing, this journey of philosophy and wisdom is led by Black women. In "Out of Racism, The Scholar" by Linda Goler Blount, chapter 2 focuses on the state of BGWH and is an ode to the scholarship on BGWH, serving as a foreword for this edited collection. In chapter 3, "BlackGirl Wellness," Dr. LeConté J. Dill uses narrative and poetry to offer the academic lineage of the term "Blackgirls" and the path to wellness. Breya Johnson anchors radical love as a health intervention to self-healing and resistance in chapter 4: "The Utility of Love for Black Women's Health." In Chinyere Okafor's (chapter 5) "The Stories We Hold: Health Implications of Embodied Narratives of Black Women and Girls from the Ivory Tower," we examine the educational system as a production of Black women's knowledge as a contribution to health. Chapter 6, Dr. Y. Falami Devoe's "Welcome to the Kitchen Table: Where Stories and Images Center the Lived Experiences of Black Women and Their Bodies," employs poetry and Black women's knowings of our bodies to curate knowledge. Dr. Shawn Arango Ricks' "Lifting As I Climb, Resting When I Need To" (chapter 7) models the self-reflexivity required to do meaningful work that creates transformative knowledge. In chapter 8, Dr. Maryam Jernigan-Noesi's "If You Can't Relate to Me, How Can You Treat Me?": Centering Black Girls' Voices in Culturally Responsive Health Praxis, offers a framework for Black girls' health and coping strategies while reimagining a Black girls' health praxis. Dr. Afiya Mbilishaka's chapter 9, "Using the Guided Hair Autobiography for Black Women and Girls as a Health Assessment" also models a self-reflexive review of intention, spirit, and personal truths as a pathway to knowledge production. In "Breaking the Concrete Ceiling: Shifting and Stress Among Black Women in the Workplace," chapter 10, by Dr. Danielle Dickens, readers receive a deeper examination of the double consciousness and shifting that Black women experience in the workplace. Chapter 11, "Eluding the White Gaze: Sex Education for Black Girls x Black Women" by Dr. Sara Flowers, offers a history of knowledge production for healers and sex health educators as she rejects the white gaze and considers the magic of sex educators, while providing historical context and contemporary best practices of Black women–informed approaches toward healthy sex and pleasure. Dr. Maranda Ward's "Black Women Stay Fighting Structural Racism: Othermothering as Community Praxis," chapter 12, offers a new way to honor the women in our communities who keep making a way out of no way, demonstrating to us the path can be our own, unapologetically. Our future is so bright and it is evident when readers dig into my Women In Science and Health (WISH) Research and Writing Lab members, as my former students reflect on their training and preparation for work in Black girls' and women's health science in chapter 13. And, in chapter 14, the Council on Black Health's leadership, Drs. Melicia Whitt-Glover, Olivia Affuso, Jameta Nicole Barlow, Shiriki Kumanyika, as well as Tambra Stevenson share the Black Health Bill of Rights, a compass, or rather North Star for our path to optimal health for Black communities.

I hope that you open your hearts, minds, and spirits to receive this knowledge and build upon these philosophies. We need this intergenerational space for the work we have been called to do, together.

REFERENCES

Bailey, M., & Peoples, W. (2017). Articulating black feminist health science studies. *Catalyst: Feminism, Theory, Technoscience*, 3(2), 1–27.

Barajas, J. (2019, August 6). *Lessons We Can Learn from Toni Morrison*. Public Broadcasting Service. Retrieved March 11, 2022. https://www.pbs.org/newshour/arts/lessons-we-can-learn-from-toni-morrison#:~:text=Take%20me%20out%20of%20it,for%20being%2C%E2%80%9D%20she%20said

Barlow, J. N., & Dill, L. J. (2018). Speaking for ourselves: Reclaiming, redesigning, and reimagining research on Black women's health. *Meridians*, 16(2), 219–229.

Barlow, J. N., & Smith, G. P. (2019). What the health (WTH)?: Theorising southern Black feminisms in the US south. *Agenda*, 33(3), 19–33.

Barlow, J. N., & Johnson, B. M. (2021). Listen to black women: Do black feminist and womanist health policy analyses. *Women's Health Issues*, 31(2), 91–95.

Beal, F. M. (2008). Double jeopardy: To be Black and female. *Meridians*, 8(2), 166–176.

Berger, M. T. (2021). *Black Women's Health: Paths to Wellness for Mothers and Daughters*. NYU Press.

Bey, M. (2019). Black fugitivity un/gendered. *The Black Scholar*, 49(1), 55–62.

Bly, A. (2021, April 26). Slave literacy and education in virginia. In *Encyclopedia Virginia*. https://encyclopediavirginia.org/entries/slave-literacy-and-education-in-virginia.

BlackPast, B. (2012, November 16). (1977) The Combahee River Collective Statement. BlackPast.org. https://www.blackpast.org/african-american-history/combahee-river-collective-statement-1977/

Coleman, C. (2021, January 29). How literacy became a powerful weapon in the fight to end slavery. *History*. Retrieved March 11, 2022. https://www.history.com/news/nat-turner-rebellion-literacy-slavery

Collins, P. H. (2002). *Black Feminist Thought: Knowledge, Consciousness, and the Politics of Empowerment*. Routledge.

Cooper, A. J. (1892). *A Voice from the South*. Xenia, Ohio, The Aldine printing house [Web.]. Retrieved from the Library of Congress. https://lccn.loc.gov/12002877

Dunbar-Ortiz, R. (2014). *An Indigenous Peoples' History of the United States* (Vol. 3). Beacon Press.

Edwards, E. R. (2021). *The Other Side of Terror: Black Women and the Culture of US Empire*. NYU Press.

Evans, S. (2019, June). *Black Women's Historical Wellness*. http://abwh.org/2019/06/21/black-womens-historical-wellness-history-as-a-tool-in-culturally-competent-mental-health-services/

Evans-Winters, V. E., & Esposito, J. (2010). Other people's daughters: Critical race feminism and Black girls' education. *Educational Foundations*, 24, 11–24.

Guy-Sheftall, B. (1995). *Words of Fire: An Anthology of African-American Feminist Thought*. The New Press.

Collins, P. H. (2002). *Black Feminist Thought Knowledge, Consciousness, and the Politics of Empowerment.* Routledge.

Collins, P. H. (1998). *Fighting Words: Black Women and the Search for Justice.* University of Minnesota Press.

hooks, b. (1997). *bell hooks Cultural Criticism & Transformation.* Media Education Foundation. www.mediaed.org/transcripts/Bell-Hooks-Transcript.pdf Date: 1997 Date accessed: June 1, 2020.

hooks, b. (2000). *Feminism Is for Everybody: Passionate Politics.* Pluto Press.

Hurston, Z. N. (1937). *Their Eyes Were Watching God: A Novel.* J. B. Lippincott Company, & Cairns Collection of American Women Writers.

James, J., & Sharpley-Whiting, T. D. (2000). *The Black Feminist Reader.* Wiley-Blackwell.

Jones, J. (2020). Troubling dignity, seeking truth: Black feminist vision and the thought-world of black photography in the nineteenth century. *Souls*, 22(1), 32–43.

King, T. L. (2019). *The Black Shoals: Offshore Formations of Black and Native Studies.* Duke University Press.

Lorde, Audre. "The Master's Tools Will Never Dismantle the Master's House." 1984. Sister Outsider: Essays and Speeches. Ed. Berkeley, CA: Crossing Press. 110-114. 2007. Print.

Maparyan, L. (2012). *The Womanist Idea.* Routledge.

Morrison, T. et al. (1975, May 30). Portland State, Black Studies Center public dialogue. Pt. 2. Series: Public Dialogue on the American Dream Theme. Retrieved from https://soundcloud.com/portland-state-library/portland-state-black-studies-1?fbclid=IwAR1eh1xHKqm3zvG9Y4NMAMvWkFTle4-4uFhY4dahEFJQUrA2wCwjLVtwBNc

Phillips, L. (2006). *The Womanist Reader: The First Quarter Century of Womanist Thought.* Routledge.

Preston, A. M. (2018). Effective allyship: A transgender woman's take on intersectionality. *Ted Talk.* Retrieved March 11, 2022. https://www.ted.com/talks/ashlee_marie_preston_effective_allyship_a_transgender_woman_s_take_on_intersectionality_jan_2018

Randolph, S. M. (2017). Evelyn Brooks Higginbotham, the metalanguage of race, and the genealogy of black feminist legal theory. *Signs: Journal of Women in Culture and Society*, 42(3), 621–628.

Schwartz, M. J. (2010). *Birthing a Slave: Motherhood and Medicine in the Antebellum South.* Harvard University Press.

Smithsonian American Art Museum. Literacy as freedom. Retrieved March 11, 2022. https://americanexperience.si.edu/wp-content/uploads/2014/09/Literacy-as-Freedom.pdf

Somé, S. (1997). *The Spirit of Intimacy: Ancient African Teachings in the Ways of Relationships.* Sobonfu Some.

Sullivan, G. (2010). Plantation medicine and health care in the Old South. *Legacy*, 10(1), 3.

Taylor, U. (1998). Making waves: The theory and practice of Blackfeminism. *The Black Scholar*, 28(2), 18–28.

Walker, A. (2004). *In Search of Our Mothers' Gardens: Womanist Prose*. Houghton Mifflin Harcourt.
Warren, C. L. (2017). Black mysticism: Fred Moten's phenomenology of (black) spirit. *Zeitschrift für Anglistik und Amerikanistik*, 65(2), 219–229.
Williams, B. C. (2018). *The Pursuit of Happiness: Black Women, Diasporic Dreams, and the Politics of Emotional Transnationalism*. Duke University Press.

Chapter 2

Out of Racism, The Scholar

Linda Goler Blount

HOW BLACK WOMEN DEFINE HEALTH

Black women are keenly aware of their health. In fact, we think about our health every day. We have to. Our thoughts may not take the form of wondering about specific diseases or whether it's time for a routine screening or even if that pain we're feeling needs to be examined. Our thoughts generally revolve around what threat, insult, or abuse we're likely to face. Whether at work, while shopping or even seeking healthcare, we know we can expect to be disrespected, disregarded, and dismissed often by well-meaning individuals. So every day, we put on our armor, gird ourselves, and prepare to face another insult while trying to care for our families, educate ourselves, earn a living, or practice self-care. And we think about what all of it means for our bodies, our minds, and our future.

In 2014, the Black Women's Health Imperative conducted a survey of Black women to understand what health meant to them. Between March 2014 and December 2017, we collected responses from 4,744 Black women on how they defined health. We collected 2,903 responses through Facebook, Twitter, and email. We attended meetings and distributed the very simple questionnaires to Black women. The questionnaire was simple: it collected name, email, age, city, and state of residency, and one question: How do you define health? There was an open-ended response line.

Eighty-five percent of all words and phrases shared were psychosocial; for example, "I'm calm," "I'm in control," "I'm at peace," and "I'm confident." Ten percent of all words and phrases were financial; for example, "I can take care of my kids," "I can keep a roof over my head," and "I can pay my bills." Five percent of all words and phrases were related to physical health and disease state; for example, "I don't have cancer," "I'm not sick," "I'm a healthy weight." We validated our results in two ways:

1) Through the Black Women's Health Study—we found that the majority of Black women self-rated their health as very good or excellent; they captured this data in their 2015 questionnaire.
2) Through social listening in 2017—we used a social media analytics tool to analyze the words Black women used to talk about health. This analysis substantiated our findings in that 80% of the words used in health discussions, postings, likes and shares were psycho-social and not specifically disease related.

To be sure, this was a convenience sample, but the number one health issue for Black women appears to be stress. Black women were telling us, "If I can get my mind right, my spirit right, and my money right, then I can take care of everything else!"

Our conclusion was that public health, policy, and clinical research practice and pedagogy that focus on Black women should start with how women feel, with what was happening to them, and with what it meant to be a Black woman in this society at this time. We should seek to understand their lived experiences and what that means not only for the health of Black women but for systems of care delivery, policies, the way we train healthcare providers, the way research is conducted, and the way we talk about data and evidence-based practices.

The authors and scholars in *Writing Black Girls' and Women's Health Science:*

Implications for Research and Praxis have known this for quite some time. Many of them have written about the lived experiences of Black women and some have conducted research to understand the impact on Black women's health and wellness. All of them have encountered barriers trying to do their work. They, too, are a part of the very same group of Black women who must put on their armor and ready themselves for daily insults. These authors, like most Black women, live at the intersection of racism and gender discrimination. Most have come to their work from economic disadvantage. And, like most Black women, they have experienced the effect of persistent stress. Research shows that Black women have on average 15% more cortisol[1] in their bloodstream at any point in time when compared with white women. We have understood the effect elevated cortisol has on the body for 30 years. In 1992, Arline Geronimus,[2] when discussing allostatic load, described the effect as weathering. She noted that Black women literally age faster than white women.

Tené Lewis found a causal relationship between experiences of racial and gender discrimination and chronically elevated cortisol which damages the DNA of Black women. Cells of the telomeres are shorter, frayed, and die sooner leaving the chromosome unprotected. This, in turn, triggers the inflammatory response as well as metabolic changes raising Black women's risk for diabetes, cardiovascular disease, certain cancers, and obesity-related syndromes. The Black Women's Health Study[3] found that if Black and white women are given the same high-fat diet, Black women will gain more weight and gain it faster; conversely, if they are given the same low-fat diet, Black women will lose less weight and lose it more slowly. And, sadly, Fleda Mask Jackson[4] found a causal relationship between stress produced by racial and gender discrimination and that produced by maternal and infant mortality. This held true particularly for well-educated, high-income-earning Black women.

Despite this research, healthcare providers blame Black women for their obesity, diabetes, and heart disease. When researchers and epidemiologists present health data by race, ethnicity, and gender, rarely do they account for or include the historical oppression and discrimination that contribute to the data they report. This is because rarely do studies include Black women or account for the historical oppression and discrimination they face.

In this book, the authors seek to connect ontology and epistemology with the understanding of how health, data, race, and gender are discussed in science, medicine, and public health. Importantly, they examine how research is conducted and how what we know as evidence is created. Despite 250 years of enslavement and 100 years of legalized oppression, the Black Women's Health Study has been the only longitudinal study to look at the epigenetic effects of historical trauma on Black women's health. The authors and scholars in this book understand how Black women view their health, the challenges they face, and that the way data are reported in no way defines who we are. *Writing Black Girls' and Women's Health Science: Implications for Research and Praxis* changes and clarifies the narrative on the health and wellness of Black women.

WHY THIS BOOK? WHY NOW?

Black women scholars have been writing about health and wellness, equity and inequalities, and racism and oppression for decades. *Writing Black Girls' and Women's Health Science: Implications for Research and Praxis* is the first book that brings a group of writers and scholars together to examine the experiences of Black women in the United States as they relate to their health. Readers will reimagine approaches to Black girls' and women's health from the perspective of philosophy and science, data, and the creation of evidence, and perhaps most importantly, interrogate how the narrative on Black women's health is developed and written.

Much of what health professionals, including clinicians, understand about Black women's health comes from studies that (1) never included Black women; (2) were derived from the abuse of Black women; and (3) assume Black women are genetically inferior to white women. Nearly all diagnostic practices for Black women are based on white women. And, when data are reported, rarely is the context of the statistic described.

For example, a much cited statistic is that Black women die at a 42% higher rate from breast cancer as compared with white women. The fact is, if Black and white women have the same breast cancer diagnosis and receive the same treatment, they will have exactly the same outcomes. In 1982, breast cancer mortality rates between Black and white women were exactly the same. There is nothing about the biologic or genetic makeup of Black women that explains the disparity in breast cancer mortality. The difference is almost entirely due to the lack of access to early detection and quality treatment. Black women simply don't have the same access as white women.

At the height of the COVID-19 pandemic, we saw multiple examples of the adverse effects of how research has been conducted in the United States and how data are used to describe Black women's health. It was discovered that pulse oximeters were not as effective[5,6] on people with dark skin complicating COVID-19 diagnoses among Black women. Dexamethasone, a steroidal treatment for lung inflammation, also was not as effective[7] among African Americans. It was later reported that no African Americans were included in the clinical trials of the drug. And, very early on in the pandemic, incidence and mortality data were not reported by race and ethnicity. It took more than six months for federal and state agencies to begin reporting disaggregated incidence and mortality data so public health officials could understand where testing resources needed to be distributed. Even armed with this data, officials were slow to get testing to Black communities. In the first eight months of 2020, Black people died at disproportionately higher rates in large part because they were less likely to have their symptoms diagnosed as COVID-19.

Provider bias in the care of Black women is, of course, well documented. We see it in HIV. Physicians are less likely[8] to prescribe HIV prevention medication to Black women because they assume they will engage in risky sexual behavior. In 2019, a study revealed that 30% of physicians believe Black people don't feel pain[9] to the same degree as white people. Sickle cell patients in pain crises, who present in the emergency department, are likely to be accused of seeking opioids and thus denied pain medication. The tragic death of Dr. Susan Moore[10,11] from COVID-19 is evidence that even Black women physicians experience provider bias—sometimes from their own colleagues.

Perhaps a less discussed issue in the literature is how the funding of research and interventional programs adversely impacts Black women. The past 35 years have been telling. Only 2% of the highest-level clinical research funds awarded by the National Institutes of Health (NIH) have gone to Black researchers. Of the research grants made by any institution to study health disparities and, particularly disparities among the Black population, over 85% have gone to white and other non-Black researchers. Private foundations, who proudly advertise their commitment to equity in health for the Black population, have routinely funded historically white-led organizations and tasked them with finding and funding Black-led community-based organizations to do the work. And, less than 15%[12] of all funds have made their way to these community-based organizations. As an example, sickle cell disease affects 100,000 Black people in the United States while there are 30,000 people living with cystic fibrosis. The funding for cystic fibrosis research and programs has been and continues to be seven times that of sickle cell disease.

The United States is at an inflection point in its history and reckoning with racism, gender discrimination, and economic oppression. More than half of all babies born are not white. COVID-19 has laid bare how systems of care delivery work against Black people and the limitations of healthcare provider training are clear. Black women are more likely to be the primary source of income in their families and demand pay equity. Black women scholars are disengaging themselves from the constraints of traditional research funding mechanisms and not only are they writing the complete truth of Black women's health, but fearlessly creating a new evidence base for Black women's health pedagogy. Black women have not been served well by evidence-based approaches to health. Our contributions to the body of literature have been devalued. And we struggle as a nation to put policies in place that would advance the health and wellness of Black women. The call to action is change: in behavior, systems, and policies.

WHAT WE CAN KNOW

In *Writing Black Girls' and Women's Health Science: Implications for Research and Praxis*, the authors aim to move medicine, public health, and the fields of social and clinical research forward by investigating the effects of omitting Black women from research and praxis. They have made recommendations for the changes in systems, behaviors, and policies required to achieve equity in the conduct of research and analysis, access to and delivery of care and, ultimately, in health outcomes. The research is clear, when the lived experiences of Black women are included in research design, program implementation, care delivery, and policy, the evidence and outcomes produced are significantly better. When they are not, the outcomes can be deadly.

On May 25, 2020, the nation watched in horror as Minneapolis police officer Derek Chauvin knelt on George Floyd's neck for 8 minutes and 46 seconds, long after Mr. Floyd complained he couldn't breathe and had stopped moving. This tragic incident was but one of 249 deaths of Black Americans that occurred at the hands of police in 2020. Given the national outrage, one might think that police killings of Black people would have decreased the following year. In fact, they increased by 6.4%.[13] We also witnessed the aftermath of the brutal shooting of Breonna Taylor in a wrong-address, no-knock warrant. In 2015, I authored an article entitled, "Can Watching Racist Viral Videos Give You PTSD?" The first paragraph begins with,

> This week, the FBI opened investigations into suspected arson at black churches in five Southern states. Last week, President Barack Obama eulogized South Carolina state Rep. Clementa C. Pinckney and other members of the Emanuel African Methodist Episcopal Church in Charleston who were shot dead June 17 as they gathered for Bible study. And three weeks ago, there was the infuriating and traumatic viral video of Eric Casebolt, a McKinney, Texas, police officer, grabbing teenager Dajerria Becton by her hair and pushing her onto the ground as she cried for her mother.

In the space of one month in June 2015, Black churches were burned, 9 black church members were gunned down, and a police officer wrestled a Black 15-year-old girl to the ground for being at a pool party. Since that article was written, more than 1,600 Black people have been killed by police, on average 1 every other day. The Anti-Defamation League[14] reported a 43%[15] rise, from 1,930 to 2,755, in the number of hate crimes against Black Americans between 2019 and 2020. Whether it is at the hands of the police, a psychopathic killer, a physician, a co-worker, or the neighbor next door, repeatedly witnessing racist acts and violence against Black people, particularly Black women, is traumatizing and our bodies respond[16] to the trauma.[17]

The authors and scholars of this book have experienced gender discrimination and racism and can attest to the effect those experiences have had on their bodies and emotional health. They write to change the way Black women are treated. This book exists so policy-makers can understand that policies born out of incompetence or racial animus must be amended if Black women are to experience health equity; so medical practice improves, providers listen to their Black patients, and their lived experiences are considered in clinical and medical technology research; so researchers and the media, when reporting health data by race and gender, acknowledge the historical racial and gender injustices that comprise the data. In doing so, they write in self-defense. They write to heal.

This book should become a part of every course on public health practice, racial and gender studies, sociology, and philosophy. It should be required reading for medical and nursing students. And no research methods course should be taught without it. I would add that courses on non-profit management and fund-raising should include this book. I would like nothing more than to have donor behavior focus on the issues and solutions put forth in this book rather than funding organizations with well-intended missions led by people who cannot understand or incorporate the lived experiences of Black women in their work.

Often when discussing racism and gender discrimination in health, providers, researchers and policy colleagues have complained to me that the subject matter is too big, too complicated—that we just can't know what to do. These two questions, *what do we need to know* and *what do we do*, have been frustratingly at the heart of much of the work and the lack of progress around Black women's health. After reading *Writing Blackgirls' and Women's Health Science:*

Implications for Research and Praxis, the answer will be clear: Now you know. Now you know how.

THE NEXT 20 YEARS

By some estimates, the year 2042 will mark a major inflection point in U.S. history. That will be the year that most adults will not be white. The majority of residents in the United States will be Black or Brown. The implications for Black women's health and wellness are significant. If we haven't achieved equity in science, health, and wealth as described in this book, then we run the very serious risk of the United States becoming pre-Mandela South Africa. Power will be concentrated in the hands of a group of people who are in the minority. Many researchers and pollsters use the term majority-minority to describe what the United States will look like in 20 years and what some states look like now. Minority is an intensely offensive term. Minority is a mathematical comparison—a person can be in the minority but not a minority.

Over the years, Black and Brown people, particularly women, have been minoritized by the use of this term. This has allowed those who are in power to overlook them for tenure, omit them from research, and not consider their needs when designing technology or therapeutics. In effect, not see them. And when Black women are not seen, they are not heard. Therefore, our complaints about feeling unwell after delivering a baby or being underpaid as compared with our white counterparts cannot be heard. We pay with our lives. The WISH Lab authors rightly point out that there must be more researchers, practitioners, department chairs, and policy-makers who look like and share the lived experiences of Black women. They will have an obvious influence on Black women's health and advancement but, as importantly, they will influence the behaviors and decision-making of those who are not Black women—of those who must see and hear Black women.

OUR IMAGINATION

The authors of *Writing Black Girls' and Women's Health Science: Implications for Research and Praxis* envision a world where Black women receive high-quality treatment by health-care providers as a matter of course, where their ideas are not only valued but sought after in academe and the workplace and, where their presence is assumed, not tolerated. In this world, the Black maternal mortality rate would be reduced significantly[18] and the gap[19] in breast cancer deaths between Black and white women would disappear. Black women represent 2.6% of all physicians—a percentage that hasn't changed in 30 years. They are less than 1% of all NIH R01 grant recipients. In 2018, Black women made up only 3% of university faculty.[20]

It is hard to say what impact equitable representation of Black women among university professorships, healthcare providers, or even corporate executives would have on society. It is fair to assume that the impact on what we consider to be knowledge, evidence, and thought would be profound. If Black women cannot participate in the development of what we consider to be evidence, then the evidence is incomplete. In their chapters, professors Okafor and Mbilishaka examine the experiences of Black women in the academy from navigating the lowered expectations of women scholars to the role hair plays in the perceptions of others about the quality of their work and thus, their career advancement. Professor Dickens points out the constant shifting required of Black women to meet and accommodate racist expectations of what is considered scholarship and thought creation takes a heavy emotional toll causing many, like Dr. Uche Blackstock,[21] to leave the work they love —often in an act of desperate self-preservation.

No research has quantified these stressors individually. In the aggregate, racism and gender discrimination are thought to contribute to nearly 100,000 premature deaths among Black people each year. The causes are many: diabetes, heart disease, stroke, cancer, among others. Dr. Jernigan-Noesi offers another powerful factor to that list: self-medication through alcohol and substance misuse. It is heartbreaking to consider where we might be as a society were it not for the thousands of brilliant people lost to the effects of racism each year.

BLACK WOMEN AT WORK

Black women in science, medicine, the academy, and in the executive ranks know that we can never be good enough. The goal posts that define success get moved with each advancement we make, and so our accomplishments often have the effect of death by a thousand cuts. We work hard, we exceed expectations, we're diminished. Rinse and repeat. Studies[22] show that where Black women experience the most racism and gender discrimination is in the workplace. This isn't surprising—most Black women between the ages of 15 and 70 work and our work, as a single activity, consumes the largest part of our day —the largest part of our lived experience, one that we depend on to keep a roof over our heads, to care for our families, to enjoy life is also the single greatest source of our stress. The workplace is perhaps the only setting where statements like "your hairstyles are always different" or "you're so dressed up" are intended not as compliments but as poisoned barbs. This dissonance of our lived experiences is revisited throughout *Writing Black Girls' and Women's Health Science: Implications for Research and Praxis*.

A well-known study[23,24] found that Black women at mid- and senior levels in for-profit corporations work on average 20% more than white women. We do so, not because that is what the work demands but because the culture of the workplace demands it. Our work is subject to intense scrutiny, second-guessing, and held to a much higher standard than that of our co-workers. The researchers noted that Black women engage in hypervigilance about their work and observed that the extra 20% that Black women work does not result in increased productivity for the company, cost-savings, or promotions. Black women double- and triple-check the accuracy and format of their work products, not because they expect constructive criticism but fault-finding. Two things are interesting about the study's findings: 1) the work products of Black women were almost always as good if not better than that of their white counterparts and, 2) if Black women were to stop working 20% more, their co-workers would not notice a difference in the quality of work or output. In other words, Black women could perform as well if not out-perform their peers working only four days per week! In *Everything But The Kitchen Sink*, Dr. Devoe adds her own experience and discusses strategies Black women can employ to protect themselves within toxic work environments.

Many of the narratives in the book refer to the kinds of improvements in health and lived experiences of Black women that would occur if more Black women were in leadership roles or valued contributors to thought. Unfortunately, this is not always the case. In follow-on surveys to the aforementioned workplace study, it has been shown that Black women work hard and are seemingly well-liked by their colleagues yet do not always enjoy continued recognition and appreciation. The so-called "Pet to Threat"[25] syndrome often derails Black women's career prospects just at the point where they should be promoted or offered a significant advance in their careers. *In Lifting As I Climb, Resting When I Need*, Dr. Ricks describes in dismay her experience in an academic setting at an HBCU and the toll on her own emotional health—the same sort of problems she encountered at primarily white institutions caused.

Black women are not monolithic, of course. We are human and have our flaws. But Dr. Ricks's experience brings to mind the work of Dr. Camara Phyllis Jones and her analysis of internalized[26] racism. It could be that Black women, even in a primarily Black academic setting, bear the brunt of the effects of internalized racism and the patriarchy of the academy. This is another perhaps, more painful, example of limits placed on Black women's contributions to science, health, and thought.

The obvious next study would be to investigate the effects working 20% more than our coworkers has on our emotional and physical health. *Writing Black Girls' and Women's Health Science: Implications for Research and Praxis* is a powerful contribution to understanding Black women's health and their contributions to science in the context of racism and gender discrimination.

Those of us who have worked in or taught public health, research, and medicine for the past 25 years have witnessed the seemingly inexorable march toward inertia. The first report on health disparities was published in 1985 by the then Secretary of Health and Human Services, Margaret Heckler. It described the disparities in health outcomes experienced by Black Americans as compared with white Americans. Since 1985, more than $200 billion has been invested in health disparities research, programs, policy analysis, and community-based interventions. By almost all measures, health disparities are worse or no better now than they were in 1985. This is certainly true for income and education inequalities.

THE WAY FORWARD

The frustration expressed by our younger colleagues is understandable. For those of us who came of age in the 60s and 70s, they wonder why we have not tapped into our inner civil rights activist, why we were not protesting that health is a justice issue, and marching in the streets in the 80s and 90s. I don't have an adequate response but I can say, many of us looked at the toll that activism took on our parents and worried about the toll it might take on us. Also, many of us had parents who insisted that a college degree, employment in good paying jobs, or as academics was the way to achieve progress for Black Americans. Some of our parents assumed that exemplary performance would result in the recognition of our skills, achievement, and promotion. They thought that perhaps by the time we were established in our careers, we might live in a meritocracy and that we would no longer need to "prove" to those in power that we were worthy of working side-by-side at the highest levels. So, many of us took that path. But we watched and listened to the generation that came after us.

They know health is a justice issue and they believe self-care is as well. In 1983, my own organization was founded on the premise and promise of self-care. It wasn't framed as a justice issue per se, but as a radical practice to deal with the injustices Black women were experiencing. Today's scholars know differently. They equate self-care, justice, and love of all of oneself. Dr. Flowers's work and research ensures Black women understand the importance and beauty of their sexual selves and the connection with health and wellness. Dr. Dill brings poetry and praxis together to prepare young Black LGBTQ scholars for the experiences they will have in the academy and to create the dependency between what we consider to be scholarship and their contributions. And, Dr. Ward has the audacity to combine justice and empathy to build community resiliency through her work to directly engage Black women in the centuries-old practice of othermothering.

The next generation knows that health is a justice issue and that justice depends on love. We owe them our full attention, mentorship, and support without prejudice. Black women must love ourselves and each other enough to get up each morning and fight for what we deserve, hold others to account, and support one another fiercely. Those of us more seasoned in this work have come to stand side-by-side our younger "sisters." We are wholeheartedly combining the more pragmatic approach we took to this work with new technologies, media, and data methods to drive change. Our research and praxis must lead to changes in behavior of corporate, health system, and academic leaders. It must lead to changes in systems of care delivery, policy development, and education.

Writing Black Girls' and Women's Health Science: Implications for Research and Praxis demonstrates the utility of love for Black women's health as Breya Johnson describes in her chapter. It also demonstrates the true collaborative spirit of intergenerational thought and scholarship—of love.

Readers of this book will observe just how hard this work is, how it wears on the authors. Sometimes it really is just too much. When that happens, out of an act of self-preservation, we must be willing and able to walk away. We must be able to count on our othermothers for help, understanding, and the grace of silence when needed. We'll come back —that's what we do.

It is my hope that *Writing Black Girls' and Women's Health Science: Implications for Research and Praxis* appears on the syllabi in public health, medical, nursing, and sociology curricula. Students in these programs must read these authors and understand how necessary Black women's contributions to research and praxis are. They must also realize the limitations of their own education and exposure. Perhaps this book will spark a thirst for more knowledge and lead to a virtuous cycle of research and collaboration among non-Black and Black scholars. This is my minimum desire for this book. The writings that follow should spark a national if not global conversation on racism, gender discrimination, and the pernicious omission of Black women from scholarship. Futurists should read this as should economists, policymakers, and business leaders. We can predict the future. *Writing Blackgirls' and Women's Health Science: Implications for Research and Praxis* helps the reader see what the lived experiences of Black women will be in 20 years if nothing changes. For those whose hands are on the levers of power, this book provides key mile markers for those who choose to make their way toward an inclusive workplace, economy, institution, and public sector. Black women will help—they already have. Our scholarship and praxis are robust and will continue. Racism and gender discrimination are not our creation nor is eliminating them our responsibility.

Read *Writing Black Girls' and Women's Health Science: Implications for Research and Praxis*, be enraged, be informed, and be inspired. Share it with your colleagues. Bring it to your classrooms. As these scholars do, envision a society without racism and gender discrimination. How would it feel? What would you do differently? Picture social media and news reports. Imagine almost no poverty, segregation, or health disparities. Visualize living in a meritocracy. That's what we do.

NOTES

1. Schreier, H. M., Bosquet Enlow, M., Ritz, T., Coull, B. A., Gennings, C., Wright, R. O., & Wright, R. J. (2016). Lifetime exposure to traumatic and other stressful life events and hair cortisol in a multi-racial/ethnic sample of pregnant women. *Stress*, 19(1), 45–52. http://doi.org/10.3109/10253890.2015.1117447

2. Geronimus, A. T. (1992). The weathering hypothesis and the health of African-American women and infants: Evidence and speculations. *Ethnicity & Disease*, 2(3), 207–221. PMID: 1467758.

3. Cozier, Y. C., Yu, J., Coogan, P. F., Bethea, T. N., Rosenberg, L., & Palmer, J. R. (April 1, 2014). Palmer, racism, segregation, and risk of obesity in the Black women's health study. *American Journal of Epidemiology*, 179(7), 875–883.

4. Jackson, F. M., Phillips, M. T., Hogue, C. J. R. et al. (2001). Examining the burdens of gendered racism: Implications for pregnancy outcomes among college-educated African American women. *Maternal and Child Health Journal*, 5, 95–107.

5. Sjoding, M. W., Dickson, R. P., Iwashyna, T. J., Gay, S. E., & Valley, T. S. (2020). Racial bias in pulse oximetry measurement. *The New England Journal of Medicine*, 383, 2477–2478.

6. https://www.fda.gov/medical-devices/safety-communications/pulse-oximeter-accuracy-and-limitations-fda-safety-communication?utm_medium=email&utm_source=govdelivery

7. https://www.hopkinsmedicine.org/news/newsroom/news-releases/steroid-drug-hailed-as-effective-covid-19-treatment-but-questions-linger-about-its-use-for-black-patients

8. Chapman, E. N., Kaatz, A., & Carnes, M. (2013). Physicians and implicit bias: How doctors may unwittingly perpetuate health care disparities. *Journal of General Internal Medicine*, 28(11), 1504–1510.

9. Hoffman, K. M., Trawalter, S., Axt, J. R., & Oliver, M. N. (2016, April 4). Racial bias in pain assessment and treatment recommendations, and false beliefs about biological differences between blacks and whites *PNAS*, 113(16), 4296-4301.

10. https://www.nytimes.com/2020/12/23/us/susan-moore-black-doctor-indiana.html

11. https://www.cnn.com/videos/us/2020/12/25/black-doctor-compains-racial-bias-covid-19-zw-orig.cnn

12. https://www.forbes.com/sites/morgansimon/2019/09/25/why-giving-your-money-away-wont-change-the-orld/?sh=23fca575b20dhttps://www.forbes.com/sites/morgansimon/2019/09/25/why-giving-your-money-away-wont-change-the-world/?sh=23fca575b20d

13. https://mappingpoliceviolence.org

14. https://www.adl.org/adl-hate-crime-map

15. https://www.adl.org/news/press-releases/adl-deeply-alarmed-by-2020-fbi-hate-crimes-data-reiterates-calls-for-increased

16. https://www.nytimes.com/2015/06/24/magazine/racisms-psychological-toll.html?smid=tw-share&_r=1

17. Williams, M. T., Malcoun, E., Sawyer, B., Davis, D. M., Bahojb-Nouri, L. V., & Leavell Bruce, S. (2014). Cultural adaptations of prolonged exposure therapy for treatment and prevention of posttraumatic stress disorder in African Americans. *Journal of Behavioral Sciences - Special Issue: PTSD and Treatment Considerations*, 4(2), 102–124.

18. Priest, N., & Williams, D. R. (2018). Racial discrimination and racial disparities in health. In B. Major, J. F. Dovidio, & B. G. Link (Eds.), *The Oxford handbook of stigma, discrimination, and health* (pp. 163–182). Oxford University Press.

19. David R. Williams PhD, MPH, Selina A. Mohammed PhD, MPH, RN, Alexandra E. Shields PhD Understanding and effectively addressing breast cancer in African American women: Unpacking the social context Cancer 29 February 2016.

20. https://nces.ed.gov/fastfacts/display.asp?id=61

21. https://fortune.com/2020/08/09/health-care-racism-black-women-doctors/

22. https://www.hsph.harvard.edu/news/press-releases/black-americans-discrimination-work-police/

23. Carter, D. R., & Peters, T. (2016). The underrepresentation of african american women in executive leadership: What's getting in the way? *Journal of Business Studies Quarterly Studies*, 7(4), 115–234.

24. https://www.shrm.org/hr-today/news/all-things-work/pages/racism-corporate-america.aspx

25. Psychological Health of Women of Color: Intersections, Challenges, and Opportunities edited by Lillian Comas-Diaz Ph.D., Beverly Greene, *Going From Pet to Threat* Kecia M Thomas, 2013.

26. https://ajph.aphapublications.org/doi/pdf/10.2105/AJPH.90.8.1212

REFERENCES

Anti-Defamation League. (August 30, 2021). ADL deeply alarmed by 2020 FBI hate crimes data; Reiterates calls for increased reporting. Retrieved from https://www.adl.org/resources/press-release/adl-deeply-alarmed-2020-fbi-hate-crimes-data-reiterates-calls-increased

Bever, L. (June 29, 2015). Five predominantly black Southern churches burn within a week; arson suspected in at least three. *The Washington Post*. Retrieved from https://www.washingtonpost.com/news/morning-mix/wp/2015/06/29/six-predominately-black-southern-churches-burn-within-a-week-with-arson-suspected-in-at-least-three/

Carter, D. R., & Peters, T. (2016). The underrepresentation of African American women in executive leadership: What's getting in the way. *Journal of Business Studies Quarterly*, 7(4), 115–134.

Chapman, E. N., Kaatz, A., & Carnes, M. (2013). Physicians and implicit bias: How doctors may unwittingly perpetuate health care disparities. *Journal of General Internal Medicine*, 28(11), 1504–1510.

CNN. (December 25, 2020). Black doctor dies of Covid-19 after accusing hospital of racial bias. Retrieved from https://www.cnn.com/videos/us/2020/12/25/black-doctor-compains-racial-bias-covid-19-zw-orig.cnn

Comas-Diaz, L., & Greene, B. (Eds.). (2013). *Psychological health of women of color: Intersections, challenges, and opportunities: Intersections, challenges, and opportunities*. Praeger.

Cozier, Y. C., Yu, J., Coogan, P. F., Behtea, T. N. Rosenberg, L., & Palmer, J. R. (April 1, 2014). Racism, segregation, and risk of obesity in the black women's health study. *American Journal of Epidemiology*, 179(7), 875–883.

Edwards, B. (June 26, 2015). Obama delivers stirring eulogy at funeral for SC state Sen. Clementa Pinckney. The Root. Retrieved from https://www.theroot.com/obama-delivers-stirring-eulogy-at-funeral-for-sc-state-1790860333

Eligon, J. (December 23, 2020). Black doctor dies of Covid-19 after complaining of racist treatment. *The New York Times*. Retrieved from https://www.nytimes.com/2020/12/23/us/susan-moore-black-doctor-indiana.html

Food and Drug Administration. (November 7, 2022). *Pulse Oximeter Accuracy and Limitations: FDA Safety Communication*. U.S. Department of Health and Human

Services. Retrieved from https://www.fda.gov/medical-devices/safety-communications/pulse-oximeter-accuracy-and-limitations-fda-safety-communication?utm_medium=email&utm_source=govdelivery

Geronimus, A. T. (1992). The weathering hypothesis and the health of African-American women and infants: Evidence and speculations. *Ethnicity & Disease*, 2(3), 207–221. PMID: 1467758.

Goler Blount, L. (July 2, 2015). Can watching racist viral videos give you PTSD? The Root. Retrieved from https://www.theroot.com/can-watching-racist-viral-videos-give-you-ptsd-1790860409

Schreier, H. M., Bosquet Enlow, M., Ritz, T., Coull, B. A., Gennings, C., Wright, R. O., & Wright, R. J. (2016). Lifetime exposure to traumatic and other stressful life events and hair cortisol in a multi-racial/ethnic sample of pregnant women. *Stress*, 19(1), 45–52. http://doi.org/10.3109/10253890.2015.1117447

Harvard School of Public Health. (October 24, 2017). Poll finds at least half of Black Americans say they have experienced racial discrimination in their jobs and from the police. Retrieved from https://www.hsph.harvard.edu/news/press-releases/black-americans-discrimination-work-police/

Hoffman, K. M., Trawalter, S., Axt, J. R., & Oliver, M. N. (April 4, 2016). Racial bias in pain assessment and treatment recommendations, and false beliefs about biological differences between blacks and whites *PNAS*, 113 (16), pp. 4296-4301.

Jackson, F. M., Phillips, M. T., Hogue, C. J. R. et al. (2001). Examining the burdens of gendered racism: Implications for pregnancy outcomes among college-educated African American women. *Maternal and Child Health Journal*, 5, 95–107.

Johns Hopkins Medicine. (June 23, 2020). COVID-19 story tip: Steroid drug hailed as effective COVID-19 treatment but questions linger about its use for Black patients. Retrieved from https://www.hopkinsmedicine.org/news/newsroom/news-releases/steroid-drug-hailed-as-effective-covid-19-treatment-but-questions-linger-about-its-use-for-black-patients

Jones, C. P. (2000). Levels of racism: A theoretic framework and a gardener's tale. *American Journal of Public Health*, 90(8), 1212.

Mapping Police Violence, Data dashboard access June 2022: https://mappingpoliceviolence.org/

Priest, N., & Williams, D. R. (2018). Racial discrimination and racial disparities in health. In B. Major, J. F. Dovidio, & B. G. Link (Eds.), *The Oxford Handbook of Stigma, Discrimination, and Health* (pp. 163–182). Oxford University Press.

Roepe, L. (February 1, 2021). Barriers for Black professionals. *SHRM*. Retried from https://www.shrm.org/hr-today/news/all-things-work/pages/racism-corporate-america.aspx

Simon, M. (September 25, 2019). Why giving your money away won't change the world. *Forbes*. Retrieved from https://www.forbes.com/sites/morgansimon/2019/09/25/why-giving-your-money-away-wont-change-the-world/?sh=23fca575b20d

Sjoding, M. W., Dickson, R. P., Iwashyna, T. J., Gay, S. E., & Valley, T. S. (2020). Racial bias in pulse oximetry measure-ment. *New England Journal of Medicine*, 383, 2477–2478.

Williams, D. R., Mohammed, S. A., & Shields, A. E. (February, 2016), Understanding and effectively addressing breast cancer in African American women: Unpacking the social context. *Cancer*. Retrieved from https://nces.ed.gov/fastfacts/display.asp?id=61

Williams, M. T., Malcoun, E., Sawyer, B., Davis, D. M., Bahojb-Nouri, L. V., & Leavell Bruce, S. (2014). Cultural adaptations of prolonged exposure therapy for treatment and prevention of posttraumatic stress disorder in African Americans. *Journal of Behavioral Sciences - Special Issue: PTSD and Treatment Considerations*, 4(2), 102–124.

Wortham, J. (June 24, 2015). Racism's psychological toll. *The New York Times*. Retrieved from https://www.nytimes.com/2015/06/24/magazine/racisms-psychological-toll.html?smid=tw-share&_r=1

Chapter 3

BlackGirl Wellness

LeConté J. Dill

A WAY WITH WORDS

In my bio that is often shared on social media, in digital spaces, and before professional and artist talks, I say that I "listen to and show up for Black-Girls and work to rigorously document their experiences of wellness." When I say *Black*, I am referring to people of African descent, African ascent (Dillard & Bell, 2011), of the African Diaspora, who identify as Black, African American, West Indian, Caribbean, Afro-Latinx, African, Blackity Black, Sho nuff Black, Hella Black, and/or Black AF. When I say *Girl*, I am referring to any cis, trans, gender-expansive, non-binary and/or any girl- or femme-identified person age 25 and younger (Grantmakers for Girls of Color, 2021), and/or who still remember or identify with their girl-hood selves. When I say *BlackGirl*, it is intentionally written as one word. I am leaning on and learning from Drs. Robin Boylorn (2016) and Dominique C. Hill (2019) who 1) reject the compartmentalization of BlackGirls' lives, stories, and bodies, 2) see the oneness of their/our identities, and 3) see them/us as whole and complex.

Now, when I say *Wellness*, well, there are a plethora of definitions, right? Especially for those of us working in and reimagining public health. For a working definition, I see wellness as being beyond illness, disease, and risk. Wellness is "beyond survival" (AAAS, n.d.). Wellness is an active pursuit of physical, mental, emotional, and spiritual safety. In Toni Cade Bambara's (1980) *The Salt Eaters*, healer Minnie Ransom asks organizer Velma Henry "Are you sure, sweetheart, that you want to be well?" (p. 3) Then Minnie goes on to say to/remind Velma "Just so's you're sure, sweetheart, and ready to be healed, cause wholeness is no trifling matter" (p. 5). So, leaning on and learning from Bambara and the healers in the fictional town of Claybourne, Georgia, wellness is also an active pursuit of one's individual and collective needs and desires. This philosophy will describe BlackGirl Wellness, situate BlackGirl Wellness as an essential part of Black Women's Health, and use ethnographic and poetic analysis to center BlackGirls as experts of their own wellness journeys.

BLACKGIRL WAYS OF BEING: BEING WELL

I come from a Chemistry Lab, flooding and on fire

I come from an English classroom snapping to fill the silence

I come from a Sociology seminar citing poets

I come from a Public Health lecture hall protesting the CDC

BlackGirl Wellness is informed by and informs public health theory and practice. Therefore, BlackGirl Wellness is bolstered by attention to the communities where BlackGirls live, learn, work, play, and pray. It understands the behaviors, relationships, organizations, and policies that work together to shape, impact, constrain, and/or support BlackGirls' lives and livelihoods. BlackGirl Wellness also understands that it is too often a missing concept, construct, and conversation in the field of public health. "Are you sure sweetheart that you want to be well?" is not found on a public health survey, interview, lecture, or conference presentation. So, BlackGirl Wellness becomes multidisciplinary, then interdisciplinary, forever transdisciplinary, perhaps antidisciplinary. BlackGirl Wellness *is* undisciplined (Sharpe, 2016)—resisting being constrained or contained, disrupting boundaries and barriers, becoming something altogether new, anew, renewed, and just being. In the poem "Black Girl Magic," poet, writer, curator, and organizer Mahogany L. Browne (2016) writes, "Black Girl they say . . . You ain't 'posed to do nothing but carry babies/And carry weaves/And carry felons . . .." Browne knows that these prevailing narratives, these "controlling images" (Collins, 1991), these tropes, these stereotypes, these assumptions are tired. Are untrue. Throughout the rest of the poem, she chants a BlackGirl anthem of excellence *and* ordinariness. The "magic" (Thompson, 2017) of Black Girlhood is a rootedness, a branching, and a blooming. Therefore, BlackGirl Wellness refutes the notion of BlackGirls and BlackGirlhoods as solely "at risk" (Dill, forthcoming). Such refutation is a clapback—BlackGirls are not too much, too little, or not enough. A BlackGirl way of being, a BlackGirl ontology, is being well.

BLACKGIRL WAYS OF KNOWING: KNOWING AND REMEMBERING BLACKGIRLS

In addition to being well, BlackGirls know wellness. A BlackGirl way of knowing, a BlackGirl epistemology, is also a BlackGirl way of knowing *and* remembering. This "know and remember" praxis comes from Saving Our Lives Hear Our Truths or SOLHOT (Brown, 2009) and invites witnesses to be in ritual to call the names, memories, and impacts of important people into a space. Rituals are inherent to Black folks—individual and collective practices of being, surviving, healing, and thriving. This is part of Black folks' spirit work, beyond religiosity (Dill, 2017); the ways of our births and our death. How we pray and play; our turn-up, our kick-back, and our wind-down. BlackGirls know and remember by asking questions: Who am I? Who My People Is (Bridgforth, 2019–present)? Who is part of the squad that I have and/or am building (Carruthers, 2018)? BlackGirls answer. BlackGirl Wellness is rememory work—recalling those memories, personal and intergenerational, tucked away (Brown, 2013; Dill, 2021; Dill, forthcoming; Dillard, 2012; Morrison, 1987). It is Sankofic–a going back to bring forward. It is remembering my and my mom's and my aunties' and my cousins' BlackGirlhoods in South Central, remembering my Nana's and her mom's BlackGirlhoods in Canfield, Arkansas, it is remembering my mama's mama's mama's mama's Black Girlhood somewhere in Alabama. It is envisioning my daughter's BlackGirlhood wherever she is alive and free. It is breathed and dreamed and danced and colored and hummed and sung and chanted and written:

They saw me dancing
I showed them how
This is the kind of love
You wish for
wait for
Told my babies
They enough
Good enough
Took them some time to see
They know now and they told you
And you found me
I knew you were coming
Home
Knew you were coming
Here (Dill, 2021)

Dear Reader, I invite you to close your eyes. Take a deep breath in, hold that breath, and take a deeper, longer breath out. Continue breathing deeply as you remember or envision your 14-year-old self. What do you see? What did you call yourself then? Call out to them! What were you proud of back then? What were you worried about? What do you know now that you wish you knew back then? Tell them! Give them some tips for their journey. Remind them that they are enough!

This BlackGirl is from South Central Los Angeles, California. South Central is one of my "homeplaces" (hooks, 1990)—a place where I was born and raised, a place from where I launched, a place where I land back; a place where I am able to be a baby bird leaving the nest, and a mama bird returning to the nest. I grew up hearing and seeing other BlackGirls from and in South Central cast to a wider audience—on airwaves, TV, and movie screens, and in magazines and newspapers. Us BlackGirls called South Central home—a blemish to some, but South Central was our blanket, our armor, our bravado, our muse, our breath. I asked for braids and beads like South Central homegirl Patrice Rushen. I wanted to be part of Yo-Yo's Intelligent Black Women's Coalition. Brandi with an "I" was one of the Girlz in the Hood and went to Spelman at the end of the movie. While Brandy with a "Y" actually went to my elementary school for a second, and you *know* everybody in L.A. knows somebody who knows somebody who is famous. And Justice wrote poetry from the ashes of the L.A. Uprising; an uprising actually sparked by Latasha . . . *or* the murder of Latasha. I have always seen Latasha as a girl, only two years older than me, who grew up not too far from me. But BlackGirls do not get to be girls. BlackGirls get to be brutes. BlackGirls get buried. BlackGirls who die too soon get buried next to their mamas who die too soon—a birthright I did not want. Latasha did not get a Sweet 16; not even a Quinceñera like our new neighbors. What to make of these rituals denied? Latasha died holding two dollars in her hand. BlackGirls are always paying. I want you to know and remember Latasha Harlins, January 1, 1976–March 16, 1991. I want you to know and remember BlackGirls beyond trauma, beyond statistics, beyond erasure, beyond hashtags for lives snuffed out. I want you to know and remember BlackGirls as nuanced, as joyful, as protected, as ordinary *and* extraordinary, as healing, as worthy.

Attending Spelman College helped me to grow my Black Feminist canon and Black Feminist praxis, which has continued to grow and to serve me throughout my life; such a joy and a privilege to learn and grow in a space that has such an enduring legacy for nurturing and bolstering BlackGirls and BlackWomxn. There, I learned (how) to call out the "matrix of domination" (Collins, 1990) and how to combat imperialist white supremacist heteropatriarchy (hooks, 1990) and also learned (more) about Black Feminists' critical role in justice movements. I did not just see Black Feminists on the bookshelf and the page, but in our classrooms, lecture halls, and auditoriums. Up close, in person, in real life. I/we learned to see Black Feminists within ourselves—19-, 20-year-old BlackGirls learning and growing and playing and partying and trying on language and conceptual frameworks and engaging in critical and radical praxes. This helped me/us to know and remember to center the sisterhood in the struggle and the joy in justice.

Black Girlhood Studies urges Black Feminists and everyone really to know and remember BlackGirls (Brown, 2009, 2013). Ladner's (1971) *Tomorrow Tomorrow*, is a pioneering sociological study of urban BlackGirls. Here is another refusal of the "Black deviance" trope. Here is a love for BlackGirls and all Black people. In 2009's *Between Good & Ghetto*, Dr. Nikki Jones asks what is the "code of the street" for BlackGirls. Here is a critical intervention across disciplines and approaches. In 2010, I asked Dr. Jones to join my dissertation committee. Through her mentoring she showed me Black Feminism-as-action, she reminded me of my Black Feminist ethnography roots nurtured at Spelman, and she made Black Girlhood Studies accessible to me and to my research participants. She remains an enduring mentor to and for me. Through SOLHOT, Dr. Ruth Nicole Brown (2009, 2013) and SOLHOT *Homegirls*, *Lil Homies*, and other crew, are in solidarity with BlackGirls to center BlackGirls across disciplines and spaces of movement work. While SOLHOT is beautifully documented across several texts by Brown and other SOLHOT Homegirls, I came to know and remember that Black Girlhood Studies is beyond the page, is enacted, is embodied, is heart work and spirit work. I am now a faculty member in a department with Dr. Brown as chairperson; a department that unapologetically centers Black Feminisms (plural)—a charge and a privilege to illuminate Black Girlhood Studies to new learners and partners and doers. I have been mentored, am being mentored, and am mentoring peers and students with a justice-based roadmap for centering BlackGirls in narratives, as knowledge producers, *and* into knowledge production. I thankfully and happily have found other BlackGirlhood ethnographers and autoethnographers along my journey, not just on the bookshelf, but on panels, conference spaces, cafes, offices, Zoom rooms, classrooms, and community spaces. Here too, up close, in person, in real life. These Black Girlhood Studies scholars, practitioners, and artists listen to, show up for, and celebrate BlackGirlhood in all of its complexities.

From 2016 to 2018, Dr. Jameta Barlow and I intentionally held space for folks to know and remember BlackGirls and BlackWomxn in and out of public health, psychology, gender and women's studies, and other disciplines. We activated a curation and reimagination of BlackGirls' and BlackWomen's Health in academic journals (Barlow & Dill, 2018), professional conferences (Barlow et al., 2017; Dill et al., 2017; Barlow, 2018), digital platforms, and community spaces. Being co-editors, co-authors, and co-moderators of such spaces is a critical intervention as two Black Feminist scholars and practitioners. It is a seeing, knowing, and remembering of other scholars, makers, and doers. It is a mentoring and nurturing in Track Changes and Comment Boxes and DMs and head nods and saying "Go Off, Sis!" when emerging and submerged scholars get the chance to testify on the page or the mic.

Such a reimagination has also paved the way for you to know and remember BlackGirl Wellness scholar-activists who are more than emerging and emergent; who are here and now and *urgent*: Dr. Mercedez Dunn,[1] Brittany Brathwaite,[2] Shanna-Kay Townsend,[3] Shavaun Sutton,[4] and Veroneque Ignace,[5] and many more named and unnamed as BlackGirl Wellness scholars, too. Specifically, #DocDillTaughtEm—it has been an honor to teach and mentor these BlackGirl scholar-activists since 2012, within and beyond the field of public health. Meeting them as practitioners and activists and scholars, and guiding and supporting them inside and outside of academic and community spaces, while centering transnational Black Feminisms and Black Girlhood Studies, has been a necessary intervention to disrupt the hegemony and epistemic violence of the public health field. And we engage in bi-directional mentoring, so my own understandings of sexual health, reproductive justice, state-sanctioned violence, the criminal legal system, the arts and health, and community-accountable scholarship have been expanded by learning from and with these scholars. Our work creates space and a spaciousness for the work of BlackGirl Health *within* the canon or subfield or inventions or conversations of Black Women's Health and public health and *outside* of it. For Black Women's Health scholars and practitioners, this calls them in, as Brown (2013) says, "to know themselves as Black girls precisely through memory and a remembered Black girlhood" (p. 51). For public health researchers and policy makers, this is more than a disaggregation of "BlackGirls" in the data; this calls in public health folks to see and recognize BlackGirls in their fullness and their complexity, to listen to them, to provide their fuller narrative, better yet, to let them narrate themselves for themselves. The praxis and pedagogy of BlackGirl Wellness is flourishing specifically because of the research, teaching, activism, and artistry of Dill, Dunn, Brathwaite, Townsend, Sutton, and Ignace.

BLACKGIRL WAYS OF DOING: WITNESSING BLACKGIRL WELLNESS

I am indebted to CEOs, executive directors, program managers, principals, teachers, staff, volunteers, and other leaders of non-profit and community-based organizations, schools, and in-school and after-school programs for inviting me to build rapport with them and inviting me into their "bird's nests" (Dill, 2015). These leaders have supported me in being a "worthy witness" (Winn & Ubiles, 2011) of their youth participants, particularly BlackGirls, over the years, over the country, and across the world. Before I conduct any ethnographic interview, I am listening to BlackGirls in a myriad of other ways. So, as a community-accountable scholar (Gumbs, n.d.) and a double dutch methodologist (Green, 2011), I may be picking up snacks, attending community meetings, teaching poetry workshops, writing letters of recommendations, assisting with grant proposals, creating policy briefs, or more, with and for the organization(s) and the young people there. I have facilitated community-engaged and community-accountable research with BlackGirls and other young people of color in East Oakland, California, Southwest Atlanta, Georgia, East Flatbush Brooklyn, New York, and Johannesburg, South Africa.

Since 2010, I have honed a method of data analysis which I have coined and published about called "participatory narrative analysis" (Dill, 2011, 2015; Dill et al., 2016, 2018). After engaging participants in ethnographic interviews about their experiences beyond illness, beyond survival, and toward wellness, I invite them back into the research space, not just as research participants, but as co-analysts of *their* data. Through a critical reading of published poetry and narrative analyses of research memos and transcripts, we have co-created individual and collective poems about navigating safety, amassing social support, and engaging in healing rituals. This is a BlackGirl way of doing—a BlackGirl methodology—of wellness. Such poetry-as-research has resulted in lesson plans, workshops, poetry chapbooks, poetry volumes, presentations, and research articles over the years. Sometimes, it has resulted in just awesome and engaging moments of calm and joy with and for BlackGirls. Overall, through this engagement and the deeper understandings that have arisen, BlackGirls know and remember themselves as co-scholars of research about and for themselves.

BLACKGIRL WAYS OF DOCUMENTING: INSIGHTS, NOT "FINDINGS," ON WELLNESS

Dr. Bettina Love (2021) reminds us that we are not "finding" out anything about BlackGirls, especially nothing that they do not already inherently know. Of course we are remembering BlackGirls. And sure, we are amplifying BlackGirl insights to more diverse venues. In this space, I want to share just a few excerpts representative of the insights that I have gleaned for more than a decade from BlackGirls, informed by BlackGirls, and about BlackGirl Wellness.

At the time of my ethnographic interviews in East Oakland, California (Dill, 2011; Dill & Ozer, 2016), LaShay (all names used are pseudonyms chosen by the girls) was 17 years old. When asked about safety in her community, she shared:

I actually stay safe by
going to school,
staying in school,
coming to work,
basically having a full schedule,
to where
I'm not just runnin' the streets

For LaShay and her peers growing up in East Oakland, staying busy, with a full schedule of activities from their waking hour until they went to sleep, is how they strategized safety in their lives and in their neighborhoods. For BlackGirls, public health's promise of "violence prevention" feels elusive. Instead, BlackGirls activate "violence management strategies" (Dill & Ozer, 2016) as they navigate safer spaces, people, relationships, organizations, and resources in their lives.

During my focus groups with middle school students in the Pittsburgh neighborhood of Atlanta, Georgia (Dill, Morrison, & Dunn, 2016), Tatiana who was 14 years old at the time, discussed safety in her community. She shared:

I always get a ride
home from school
from my family
I don't feel safe walking
home from school
cars slow down
and look at me

Although there were active "obesity prevention" initiatives in Tatiana's neighborhood at the time of data collection encouraging walking and biking to school instead of driving or riding in a car, it was often not safe to do so, especially for BlackGirls. Living in a neighborhood ravaged by the foreclosure crisis created a landscape of abandoned houses, or "bandos," fewer "eyes on the street" (Jacobs, 1961), and heightened gender and sexual violence there. Play, frivolity, or a leisurely stroll through the neighborhood was often also foreclosed upon for Tatiana and her peers. BlackGirls strategically navigate safer routes and modes of travel, particularly in their journeys between their homes and their schools.

Jay was a participant in the Kings Against Violence Initiative (KAVI) in the East Flatbush neighborhood of Brooklyn, New York when she was in high school. She was referred to the program by school administrators and teachers that often labeled her as too loud, too much, "a fighter," and "a truant." Her trauma history, her resilience, and her brilliance were too-often not recognized. I invited Jay to participate in an ethnographic interview with me (Dill, Rivera, & Sutton, 2018; Dill et al., 2019) when she was 19—a year after she graduated from high school and after her direct involvement in the program. She was able to reflect that, ". . . coming to KAVI, I think that was the first time [that] I cried. It was just like I just finally got to release and be comfortable. They were actually really supportive." Jay found a safe space where she was able to emote, not at home or in class, but through the KAVI program—surrounded by other BlackGirls with whom she was building solidarity and camaraderie and supported by BlackWomxn facilitators-as-mentors. During the preliminary analysis stage of the KAVI interviews (Dill, Rivera, & Sutton, 2018), Nidi was 15 and a current KAVI participant. She read Jay's transcripts and co-analyzed the data with me. She responds to Jay with a letter-poem:

Dear Jay,
You know the worth of yourself
Don't let nobody bring you down.
Because you are good enough!

Nidi showed Jay empathy, respect, and support, through her analytical praxes. Across geographies, BlackGirls willingly engage with poetry to unpack identities, to trouble systems and structures, and to celebrate (their) complexities. Poetry, as inquiry and analysis, are BlackGirl ways of documenting their practices of safety, which are practices and journeys of wellness.

TOWARD A PRAXIS OF BLACKGIRL WELLNESS

BlackGirl Wellness praxes may take the form of poetry, spoken word performances, and chapbooks. They may be vision boards, collages, or murals. They may be pages scribbled in a diary, or pages submitted to "peer review" to be published. They may be memes, gifs, or blogs. They may be tears, wails, whispers, shouts, screams, giggles, and guffaws. They may be prayers, chants, affirmations, asanas, or deep breaths. They may be dances, TikTok videos, songs, or selfies. BlackGirl Wellness praxes give a side-eye, throw shade, roll necks, and give dap, blow kisses, or pull in real close for a consensual embrace. BlackGirl Wellness praxes are crunk (Dill, forthcoming) *and* chill *and* the rich, liminal spaces in between. BlackGirl Wellness implores scholars and practitioners to learn how BlackGirls (already) measure, analyze, and document hope, love, and joy. To #CiteBlackGirls. To do what Mahogany L. Browne says and to "build a universe for every kind of Black girl" (Lincoln Center, 2022). Such BlackGirl Futurisms (Jarmon, 2013; Woodson, 2016)—of dreaming, of agency, of healing, of thriving—contribute to our understandings of research and praxes on the health and wellness of BlackGirls.

NOTES

1. https://news.umbc.edu/umbcs-merdecez-dunn-illuminates-marginalized-voices-to-boost-equity-from-public-health-to-the-classroom/
2. https://www.brittanybrathwaite.com/
3. https://www.linkedin.com/in/s-kaytownsend/
4. https://cssh.northeastern.edu/student/shavaun-sutton/
5. https://www.veronequeignace.com/bio--cv.html

REFERENCES

Bambara, T. C. (1980). *The Salt Eaters*. Vintage.

Barlow, J. N. (2018, May 17–19). *Re-Imagining Black Girls' and Women's Health: Symposium and Workshop*. Towson: Towson University.

Barlow, J. N., & Dill, L. J. (2018). Speaking for ourselves: Reclaiming, redesigning, and reimagining research on Black Women's Health. *Meridians: Feminism, Race, Transnationalism, 16*(2), 219–229.

Barlow, J. N., Dill, L. J., Jones, L. V., & Guy-Sheftall, B. (2017, November 16–19). Bridging the gap between disciplines to address Black Women's Health [Roundtable Session]. National Women's Studies Association Annual Conference, Baltimore. https://convention2.allacademic.com/one/nwsa/nwsa17/index.php?cmd=Online+Program+View+Session&selected_session_id=1269028&PHPSESSID=7hr0f45t120g1594konn8n3lq3.

Boylorn, R. M. (2016). On being at home with myself: Blackgirl autoethnography as research praxis. *International Review of Qualitative Research, 9*(1), 44–58.

Bridgforth, S. (Host). (2019-Present).*Who Yo People Is*. Geeched Out Productions. https://www.whoyopeopleis.com/.

Brown, R. N. (2009). *Black Girlhood Celebration: Toward a Hip-Hop Feminist Pedagogy*. Peter Lang.

Brown, R. N. (2013). *Hear Our Truths: The Creative Potential of Black Girlhood.* University of Illinois Press.

Browne, M. L. (2016). *Black Girl Magic*. New York: Roaring Book Press.

Carruthers, C. (2018). *Unapologetic: A Black, Queer, and Feminist Mandate for Radical Movements*. Beacon Press.

Collins, P. H. (1990). *Black Feminist Thought: Knowledge, Consciousness, and the Politics of Empowerment*. New York: Routledge.

Collins, P. H. (1991). Controlling images and Black women's oppression. *Seeing Ourselves: Classic, Contemporary, and Cross-Cultural Readings in Sociology, 4,* 266–273.

Department of African American and African Studies. (n.d.). *About.* Michigan State University. https://aaas.msu.edu/about/.
Dill, L. J. (2011). *Routes to Resilience: Mechanisms of Healthy Development in Minority Adolescents from High-Risk Urban Neighborhoods* (Doctoral dissertation). UC Berkeley School of Public Health, Berkeley, CA. http://escholarship.org/uc/item/8516552z.
Dill, L. J. (2015). Poetic justice: Engaging in participatory narrative analysis to find solace in the "Killer Corridor". *American Journal of Community Psychology, 55*(1–2), 128–135.
Dill, L. J. (2017). "Wearing my spiritual jacket": The role of spirituality as a coping mechanism among African American youth. *Health Education & Behavior, 44*(5), 696–704.
Dill, L. J. (2021). Breathe into Believing. *Hypatia, 36*(3), 555–565.
Dill, L. J. (2022). Maroons: Blackgirlhood in Plain Sight. *Feminist Anthropology, 3*(2), 263–273.
Dill, L. J. (2023). #CrunkPublicHealth: Decolonial feminist praxes of cultivating liberatory and transdisciplinary learning, research, and action spaces. In J. Ford & N. Jaramillo (Eds.), *Disrupting Colonial Pedagogies: Theories and Transgressions* (pp. 115–133). Champaign: University of Illinois Press.
Dill, L. J., Barlow, J. N., Jones, L. V., Ignace, V., Dixon Diallo, D., Brathwaite, B., Huggins, K., Myles, R., Roberts, L., Jolly, J., & Harris, F. (2017, November 4–8). *African American Women's Health Across the Life Span* [Roundtable Session]. American Public Health Association Annual Meeting, Atlanta, GA. https://apha.confex.com/apha/2017/meetingapp.cgi/Session/51024.
Dill, L. J., Morrison, O., & Dunn, M. (2016). The enduring Atlanta compromise: Black youth contending with home foreclosures and school closures in the "New South". *Du Bois Review: Social Science Research on Race, 13*(2), 365–377.
Dill, L. J., & Ozer, E. J. (2016). "I'm not just Running' the Streets" exposure to neighborhood violence and violence management strategies among urban youth of color. *Journal of Adolescent Research, 31*(5), 536–556.
Dill, L. J., Rivera, B., & Sutton, S. (2018). "Don't let nobody bring you down": How Urban Black girls write and learn from ethnographically-based poetry to understand and heal from relationship violence. *The Ethnographic Edge, 2*(1), 57–65.
Dill, L. J., Sutton, S., Rivera, B., & Amory-Powell, A. (2019). "I can only do me": African American, Caribbean American, and West African girls' transnational nature of self-articulation. In J. Jordan-Zachery & D. Harris (Eds.), *Black Girl Magic: Beyond the Hashtag* (pp. 60–79). Tucson: The University of Arizona Press.
Dill, L. J., Vearey, J., Oliveira, E., & Castillo, G. M. (2016). "Son of the Soil . . . Daughters of the Land": poetry writing as a strategy of citizen-making for lesbian, gay, and bisexual migrants and asylum seekers in Johannesburg. *Agenda, 30*(1), 85–95.
Dillard, C. B. (2012). *Learning to (Re)member the Things We've Learned to Forget: Endarkened Feminisms, Spirituality, and the Sacred Nature of Research and Teaching*. New York: Peter Lang.

Dillard, C. B., & Bell, C. (2011). Chapter twenty-one: Endarkened feminism and sacred praxis: Troubling (auto) ethnography through critical engagements with African indigenous knowledges. *Counterpoints, 379*, 337–349.

Grantmakers for Girls of Color. (2021). *Theory of Impact Statement*. https://grantmakersforgirlsofcolor.org/wp-content/uploads/2021/07/G4GC-THEORY-OF-IMPACT-June-FINAL-VERSION.docx-2.pdf.

Green, K. (2011). Doing double dutch methodology: Playing with the practice of participant observer. In D. Paris & M. Winn (Eds.), *Humanizing Research: Decolonizing Qualitative Inquiry with Youth and Communities* (pp. 147–160). Los Angeles: Sage.

Gumbs, A. P. (n.d.). Brilliance Remastered. http://www.alexispauline.com/brilliancerremastered.

Jacobs, J. (1961). *The Death and Life of Great American Cities*. New York: Random House.

Jarmon, R. (2013). *Black Girls Are from the Future: Essays on Race, Digital Creativity, and Pop Culture*. Washington, DC: Jarmon Media.

Jones, N. (2009). *Between Good and Ghetto*. Rutgers University Press.

Hill, D. C. (2019). Blackgirl, one word: Necessary transgressions in the name of imagining Black girlhood. *Cultural Studies? Critical Methodologies, 19*(4): 275–283.

hooks, B. (1990). *Yearning: Race, Gender, and Cultural Politics*. Boston: South End Press.

Ladner, J. (1971). *Tomorrow's Tomorrow: The Black Woman*. Garden City: Doubleday.

Lincoln Center. (2022, January 11). *Book Release Reading: Vinyl Moon by Mahogany L. Browne* [Video]. YouTube. https://www.youtube.com/watch?v=G6lD8tIDbi8.

Love, B. (2021, January 27). *Abolitionist Teaching: A Conversation with Bettina L. Love*. Evanston: Northwestern University.

Morrison, T. (1987). *Beloved*. New York: Knopf.

Sharpe, C. (2016). *In the Wake: On Blackness and Being*. Durham: Duke University Press.

Thompson, C. (2017). *Black Girl Magic*. https://medium.com/@thepbg/a-long-long-time-ago-on-a-blog-far-far-away-i-once-wrote-about-what-black-girl-magic-means-to-me-c4642e4f2f96.

Winn, M. T., & Ubiles, J. R. (2011). Worthy witnessing: Collaborative research in urban classrooms. In A. Ball & C. Tyson (Eds.), *Studying Diversity in Teacher Education* (pp. 295–308). New York: Rowman and Littlefield.

Woodson, J. (2016). *Brown Girl Dreaming*. Penguin.

Chapter 4

The Utility of Love for Black Women's Health

Breya Johnson

BLACK READING TO HEAL: THE UTILITY OF LOVE FOR BLACK WOMEN'S HEALTH

Philosophy of Science

I must begin this chapter by locating myself in this dialogue and in this material world as a Black feminist and womanist scholar—whose intellectual formation is constructed through a lens of abolition, psychoanalysis, Black psychology, and reproductive justice. I owe a good amount of my political consciousness-raising to the organizing efforts around the murders of Trayvon Martin, Aiyana Stanley-Jones, and Sandra Bland. I owe my understanding of praxis to the reproductive justice movement and radical workers throughout the care economy. I owe much of my personal radicalization to the writings of Black women, various liberation movements throughout the global south, and my experience as a student organizer at Towson University for #Occupy-Towson. Using the writings of Black women to guide my praxis and support my healing has always been my philosophy because so much has already been written for us to return to. It is the literal writings, the reading of the texts, and the memory work all together that serve as a healing modality for Black women's health. Building on these modalities that are materialist, Black feminist, and concerned with Black women's inner workings helps us reorder ourselves. The practice of honoring what we know and how we feel so much that we write it down is imperative. This is memory work and remembrance.

Introduction

Living through major socio-political andcultural moments as a young Black woman and my interpersonal experience thrusted me into a deep concern for

Black health and well-being. Throughout my undergraduate tenure, I grew increasingly interested in what I began to call the "pedagogy of disposability"—the belief that the messages from society that make up the fabric of our institutions are structurally and culturally designed to teach people that they are disposable. Moreover, they are constructed to erase and delegitimize the lives of the marginalized, the subaltern, and the vulnerable. Modes of disposability impact the inner workings of Black women. I am deeply concerned with how "imperialist white-supremacist capitalist patriarchy" (hooks, 2010) vehemently attacks the self-confidence, self-actualization, and material reality of Black people. It disrupts our ability to love in all forms. This has detrimental effects on the health of Black women. I am most interested in the inner workings of Black women—depression, grief, pain, stress, confusion, madness, and more that show up in our bodies and health outcomes. We have data that reveals living under systems of domination causes a weathering of the body and spirit. Our weathering is reflected in maternal outcomes, chronic disorders, blood pressure, anxiety, depression, and more.

After the ancestral transition of our beloved foremother Toni Morrison in 2019, I found myself revisiting her words and her love for us. What sits in my heart and compels me the most is her call on us to love our flesh because *she loved us that much.* Love your flesh — the highest honor and our greatest call to action as Black women. I first discovered Morrison and her radical writings in high school, at that time I did not understand how political this personal call was. After the ancestral transition of bell hooks in 2021, I found myself in deep grief because she was largely responsible for my radicalization around love and care. As my Black Feminist Consciousness started to develop her work gave me the language I was searching for. What I loved about the writings of Black women was how they instantly affirmed that aching that was within them and me. The type of ache you have as a young person because you know something is wrong, you are dissenting or seeking to dissent before you even know what that word means. You don't know just yet that Black feminisms is about a practice of dissent and refusal. You are frustrated and curious about the world. And in some cases, you feel alone or isolated in your pain.

But, then, you read.

You read that first text written by a Black woman or radical Black writer and you are gifted *language.* Language that helps you understand who you are and what is happening to you, language that contextualizes the world, language that passes down community praxis and knowledge. You are able to remember. When you write you are able to release, remember, and find a location for healing.

Contextualizing Radical Love/Love-Politics

Black Feminists and Womanists have long theorized about romantic relationships or love in general; many refer to this now as love-politics (I prefer to call it radical love), where love is said to be deeply embedded in our movements, community, and radical action. The Combahee River Collective statement declared that their actions came from a "healthy love of themselves and their community." Toni Morrison and Alice Walker have written extensively about abusive relationships in the Black community. Anna Julia Cooper, Ntozake Shange, Audre Lorde, Patricia Hill Collins, Nina Simone, and bell hooks have been grappling with the love of themselves, community, and romantic partners through scholarship and art. In fact, Jennifer Nash defined "black feminism's pleas for love as a significant call for ordering the self *and* transcending the self, a strategy for remaking the self *and* for moving beyond the limitations of selfhood" (Nash, 2013).

During the late 1960s and early 1970s Black Feminist and Black power movements, there was a political necessity to practice radical love. Black Feminists theorists were overwhelmingly proponents of radical humanism, committed to the love and liberation of all people. The love of people and the community served as the dominant and radicalizing discourse for organizing. "It is our duty to fight for our freedom. It is our duty to win. We must love and support one another. We have nothing to lose but our chains." was Assata Shakur's way of articulating a political strategy deeply invested in what we now know as love-politics. The "fight" and "win" are a *duty* but "love" is a *must*. The Combahee River Collective statement was also an articulation of love; many scholars have named this as the birthplace of identity politics. However, what has been neglected or undervalued was their claim that "our politics evolve from a healthy *love for ourselves, our sisters, our community which allows us to continue our struggle and work*." This was an accountable sustainable love that will work in service of the entire community. The use of language here is a strong indication that it is within that love, one is able to engage in radical social justice work. That love is a catalyst. To the collective love is "healthy," they have set an important criterion on the love that reveals transcending the self and moving away from undefined vague ideas of love. Joy James defines revolutionary love as "difficult to define, district from personal or familial love, it originates from a desire for the greater good that entails radical risk-taking for love.". Distinct from personal or familial love, it originates from a desire for the greater good that entails "radical risks taking for love" (James 2022). James raises the stakes and moves us toward an understanding of love that moves beyond the charming or romantic notions of love so that we can understand risks taking is an essential part of the work.

Alice Walker has spent decades expressing the importance of love in what is arguably the private and public sphere. She has been relentless in her assertion that self-love is a critical component to everything in life, in her definition of womanism, Walker, says a womanist "loves herself regardless." The "regardless" being positioned last is a clear indication of its necessity. She does not leave room for a "but" or "maybe," nothing is allowed to negate that self-love because it is mandatory. Walker published *Anything We Love Can be Saved*; the title illuminates the inability to separate the private and public spheres with regard to love. To Walker in order to save oneself or the world we have to begin with self-love. For Walker, love is a strategy of orienting the self away from the frivolous, from the insignificant, and toward what she describes simply as the "serious" (Nash, 2013). Walker's most famous novel *The Color Purple* relentlessly focuses on Black women's vulnerability. We witness a Black woman learn to love herself "regardless" even though the sexual, physical, and emotional abuse was imposed upon her by those who were supposed to love her. Moreover, it was the act of loving herself and loving her sister, and loving another woman sexually and emotionally that compelled her to leave that violent space called home.

The act of loving herself is what Walker strategically shows led to her liberation. Walker shifted cultural ideas of who is worthy of love. Toni Morrison (2008) was interviewed on her motivation for writing in the mid-1960s; she claimed: "most of the publications during that time had a very powerful, aggressive, revolutionary fiction or nonfiction with a very positive racially uplifting rhetoric to go with it." Morrison was concerned that these affirmations would cause them to skip over something critical. She says, "Before we all decide that we are all beautiful and have always been beautiful, let me speak for some of us who didn't get that right away." Again, we must focus on those feelings. Alice Walker and Toni Morrison use writing to move away from acts of love that neglect dealing with the most painful parts of the self. *Instead, they force us to examine modes of love, how love is contested, dispersed, and made sensible.*

Nina Simone articulated in her interview on Blackness, that she felt compelled to push young Black people to identify with Black culture. Simone claimed that her "job is to get them (Black people) or pursued them by hook or crook to get more aware of themselves and where they came from. . . . and I will do it by any means necessary." This deliberate goal of hers is made evident in all of her music as she champions blackness as beautiful and resilient. She radicalizes Black people through music and participates in the Black Power movement through her artistry. Simone was compelled to use music and love to do her part in Black liberation. Walker and Simone share in the fundamental idea that the love of the self is critical, as it leads to an understanding of the self that then serves as a catalyst for radical action and a type of radical humanism. In her song *The Look of Love,* Simone asserts: "That love is the only thing worthwhile/There'll be music for everyone." In order for the entire world to smile, there must be a consensus on the importance and transformative power of radical love. When talking about love in the public sphere, there is always an affirmation that incites one to rise up for a cause. This is another location where radical action can be made possible as people leap into radical direct action work. We need the cause to be in service of the Radical Black Feminist and Womanist tradition and it is my vision.

Grappling with the various forms of love is embedded in Black Feminist and Womanist scholarship. Each writer or artist mentioned above was using their understanding of love to push Black people toward a political goal. This does not mean that we all agree on the end goal or even share the exact same definitions of love, but rather, we all find some kind of utility in examining or trending to love. "We want the feminist goal that the personal is political to illuminate all of our choices" (Nash, 2013).

In her essay *Practicing Love: Black feminism, Love-Politics, and Post-Intersectionality* Nash (2013) provides a more recent assessment and overview of Black women writers grappling with love and all its political implications. Her most notable assessment was on Alice Walker's *In Search of Our Mothers Garden;* where she defines womanism and self-love:

> Walker's plea for self-love articulates a relationship between self and politics, revealing that womanist politics requires a particular orientation of self, and that ethical management of the self might even *prefigure* the political and creative projects that the womanist subject engages in. womanist politics requires subjects to work on themselves in order to transcend their selves; it is, then, a radical articulation of the political limitations of selfhood. (Nash, 2013)

Another major contribution to this growing theoretical conversation on love Nash made was her conclusion that love-politics does the work intersectionality has failed to do:

> In describing intersectionality as present-oriented, I do not mean to deny intersectionality's commitment to a just social world, which is, of course, a visionary project, or to discount its normative project: reconfiguring legal doctrine, insisting on the inherent value of black women's experiences, reformulating feminist and antiracist theory. What I mean, though, is that intersectionality relies on an attachment—perhaps even a cruel attachment—to the present in two ways: first, it insists that redress can be crafted *within the confines* of the social moment as it now exists. Legal doctrine can be reformed to make cognizable race-*and*-gender-based discrimination claims; feminism can be recrafted to "include" black women's experiences; antiracist work can be transformed to take seriously black women's injuries. Second, intersectionality's very conception of identity, which treats race and gender as fixed, coherent, and legible, "presupposes identity and

> thus disavows futurity, or, perhaps more accurately, prematurely anticipates and thus fixes a permanence to forever" Although intersectionality fixes identity, presuming that race and gender are stable categories that interact in particular and knowable ways, it also aspires to make visible those identities and their intersections in the "here-and-now." (Nash, 2013)

Instead of doing this, love-politics reimagined a world ordered by love, embracing radical difference, with subjects who work on themselves to work for each other.

There is no place for intentional harm in love, and if we want systemic harm to end, we have to become more intentional about the manner in which we love and our imagery on love. Love is only easy to weaponize and manipulate when you do not have a value-informed definition of love. I remain suspicious of those who use love to replace power and replicate systems of domination onto others in the name of loving them. Like Toni Morrison, I am weary of those who leap at the idea of affirmative love without taking time to sit in the despair of hating oneself and processing that pain. I am most interested in a kind of radical love that is indicative of the fact that we cannot separate the private and public sphere. Love that makes us all deeply interrogate the harm we have caused and the harm we have felt in order to minimize causing harm moving forward for radical risk taking. At this time, I find Joy James's definition of revolutionary love to have the most potential.

Black Health and Healing Praxis

Contextualizing radical love is important to this healing modality because in a quest to trace a theory of love present in Black writings, what I found was attempts Black women made throughout history to move us into caring and loving each other, healing, and fighting back against anti-black systems of domination that render us unwell. In the terrain of these writings I received recipes for my own healing and I started writing back to those recipes, creating my own and cooking them up in my own life for deeper nourishment.

bell hooks work helped me reimagine health for Black people. I started to make a serious connection between how I was caring for myself and how the outside world informed that quality of care. Understanding my relationship to being a caregiver was one of the most intimate ways I was able to understand my family dynamics and my relationship to the state. In *Sisters of the Yams: Black Women and Self Recovery,* hooks states that Black women's passive acceptance of being omnipotent caregivers is a barrier to self-recovery. Even caretaking contributes to the weathering health of Black women. Morrison helped me love myself but hooks revealed a more expansive conception of love. Her work refused to turn away from pain. She provided an understanding of love that pushed back against everything dominant culture teaches us. A collectivist love approach that has changed the lives of so many Black women. How do we undertake her work on love and healing to shift the reality of Black women's health? This revived my motivation to explore the utility of love even more beyond the limitations of romance of selfhood.

As I was having that experience in literature my own lived experience started to show me the directions I needed to move toward. Some years doing organizing work and being a college student had taken a tremendous toll on my body. I still have a memory of being in my campus health center for dehydration and pulling an IV out of my arm so I could attend a rally on campus. I reflect on that moment all the time. The years I have spent doing survivor support, research, organizing, all while attending school and working. I did it all through chronic headaches, isolation, severe stomach issues, and more. I may never feel fully comfortable revealing what campus organizing did to my body. But, I hold on to the writing that helped me move through those moments. I knew what I was doing was unsustainable but I needed both ancestral and communal support to get off that hamster wheel. This looked like on campus "sister circles" and reading Audre Lorde's "The Cancer Journals." My great-grandmother on my mother's side of the family died of breast cancer before I was born and sitting with Audre's raw accounts on her experience with the same health crisis was both devastating and a sense of recovery for me. I learned more about Black women's health and I wonder what aspects of Audre's experience were similar to my great-grandmother's. I put that text down feeling like I had a better understanding of cancer, which before just felt like the boogeyman—something so many women in my family have survived or died from that you were just supposed to "pray" never happens to you or anyone else you love. Another moment was the power of reading and writing as memory work became clearer to me.

Like many Black women I was hurting, I felt unbearable pain about the reality of my health and the health of people I loved. Witnessing them navigate their own health as Black women is one of the biggest reasons that I give this work my life. Lupus, cancer, diabetes, asthma, depression, anxiety, PTSD, and more are all health concerns the women I love most in the world have had to hold. I started to wonder how much of this was a result of trapped emotions. Our bodies are holding feelings about isolation and despair. Much of what I saw in my own body was the result of those things. I understand fully that anti-Black world is responsible for this; however, my focus is on what we do in spite of this world. There I was with organizing experience, a deep commitment to Black feminist writings, and my own lived experience, three things that would make up my approach to Black health. There were three things that felt like facts to me:

1. Abolition also means hospitals—The healthcare industry must also be understood as an extension of carceral practices. A site of disposability for Black women.
2. The inner workings of Black women matter—feelings, trapped emotions, pain must be centered.
3. Love has utility—what are the care practices we can dream up as healthcare systems continue to fail us?

Abolition: The fall of *Roe v. Wade* has forced many people to confront the collaboration between healthcare and police/prisons. As more states continue to ban abortions, we now have all our reproductive care under more intense threats of violence. If healthcare providers are mandated reporters that would mean even the most ethical of them will still have to cooperate with the state. America has always found ways to criminalize reproductive care. Many healthcare providers enact violence upon Black people. I'm less invested in regurgitating the same statistics that prove the non-care we receive from medical professionals that leads to trauma and/or premature Black deaths. I am invested in folks seeing these professionals as collaborators in the project of anti-blackness. I envision our movement going in a direction where we protest and engage in direct action against hospitals, big pharma, and healthcare providers with the same tenacity we give police brutality. Instead of bombarding our communities with the statistics about negative outcomes that are only being internalized and causing more fear, we need to push them closer to trusting in our ability to create better systems of care. As an abortion doula, I have to constantly remind people that western practitioners are not the only experts. In my time as an organizer, I have seen birth, death, grief, and abortion doulas learn lifesaving skills and bring that knowledge back to their communities. In 2020, the police murders of George Floyd and Breonna Taylor caused major uprisings all across the states. This political moment of Black resistance brought "aboliton" into mainstream conversations and the phrase "defund the police" became a source of major political tension and debate. The demand was to defund the police and fund communities, organizers offered up funding housing, education, public transit, child care, elderly care, and healthcare. I noticed that many people named community health centers and universal healthcare as a major need, which is of course true. The disconnect is when you take a closer look at what systems they were offering up as places for the police dollars to go as we continue to prioritize western systems of care. We need to fund all doulas, abortion funds, street medics, harm reduction practitioners, and more. Western knowledge and healthcare practices are not the only way.

Inner Workings: In my time as an organizer, I found myself in constant debates with my comrades about healing and therapy. I will never forget someone saying to me that our communities needed resources not therapy. Or, how talking about personal healing was met with hostility or pivoted to conversation about the next direct action. I learned quickly that many people see these things in a binary. We do absolutely need resources and therapy alone isn't the answer but I will never concede to the idea that our inner work and political resistance should not both be a priority. We have to understand political education as a process of doing inner work. Consciousness raising can be a healing methodology as we shift peoples' understanding of the problem, the world, and move them closer to our respective causes. I have also witnessed organizers work themselves into destruction because they spent so much time only politicizing and theorizing their way out of their emotions. I know far too many organizers who can tell you exactly what's wrong in their communities, they can cite all the sources, they can propose solutions, and testify for or against any city council initiative but they cannot sit with their own emotions worth a damn. And for many Black people, seeking professional mental healthcare will never be an option by choice because of its relationship to carcerality. Self-help books would not be such a money maker if our communities were not desperately seeking ways to heal.

Love's Utility: When I think about the utility of love, I think about what it means to expand our capacity to care. As suffering continues and intensifies most people will reduce their caring capacity and pivot to only thinking about themselves. This isn't inherently malicious, when our lives or the world implodes, all we can do is take care of ourselves. However, it is up to us as practitioners and organizers to push people in caring for each other because it is the only way we will survive the fascist attacks and ecological crisis we are living in. We know people are stuffing and it only benefits the state when we focus on our sole survival. We all rely on care to survive. According to the American Psychiatric Association's *Mental Health Facts for African Americans* guide, they are also: Less likely to receive consistent care, less frequently included in research, and more likely to use emergency rooms or primary care (rather than mental health specialists). These alarming facts make the work of Black feminists like bell hooks an imperative because she drew connections between health, self- recovering, and political resistance. It is up to us to care for Black people by utilizing love in ways that refuse domination and/or neglect.

Again, our current political landscape is intensifying suffering: The Supreme Court has overturned abortion protections, LGBTQ protections, and affirmative actions. The court has denied student loan debt relief. We have record-breaking levels of air pollution and other environmental degradation. We are in year three of the Covid-19 pandemic. And rates of violence, especially against women and marginalized genders, are increasing. Abortion funds are running out of money. And evictions are rising. Lastly, it is clear that many Black women are in deep pain. That they are struggling with overwhelming feelings of despair and grief. Suicide is a silent crisis among Black women. The most recent CDC data available suggest that, suicide rates among white people in the United States declined from 2019 to 2020. But there were no statistically significant declines in suicide rates for Black Americans. The suicide rates of Black youth and young adults have steadily increased over the last 20 years. So where does that leave Black women who are holding so much? Where can Black women go when they are overstimulated, depressed, grieving, and/or traumatized? (This fundamental question would lead me toward the work I do today.) Our community still doesn't know how to love Black women who are struggling mentally and emotionally.

We have to love each other in a way that serves as a health invention. I am of the Black feminist genealogy that believes we must enact radical love and care on ourselves and on our community. Some of these self-reflexive engagement inquires:

- How long have you been in pain?
- What are your earliest memories of grief and suffering?
- Did anybody teach you where to put that pain or how to get it out of your body?

These are questions that motivate my approach to Black women's health. My approach is one of love—a care ethic that compels us to refuse individualism. There is no future where individualism will be sufficient. Capitalism has socialized us into this failed project of individuals but we have to remember that only collectivist approaches will push us into a healthier reality. My care-ethic is an approach that centers our internal longings, self-perception, and ability to love. An approach that prioritizes how we feel and move through deep rooted grief and trauma that we have inherited. An approach that teaches us how to care for Black women with mental health concerns as opposed to disappearing them into hospitals or completely neglecting them. My time in movement has taught me a lot of care planning, pod mapping, and communal approaches.

Black Reading to Heal

In an attempt to draw connections between abolition, Black women's inner workings, and love, I had to go into the archives. In my years of doing research and writing I noticed the positive impact it was having on me. I wasn't just learning, I was healing. In an attempt to provide healing and political education I started the blog Black Reading to Heal. Reviving the work of Black women writers is my approach with my work at Black Reading to Heal—in this work I find locations and mechanisms for healing. Every reading offers a way of knowing and being unique to Black women. bell hooks understood the transformative power of theory in her essay *Theory for Liberatory Practice* (1991) when she writes:

> Let me begin by saying that I came to theory because I was hurting-the pain within me was so intense that I could not go on living. I came to theory desperate, wanting to comprehend-to grasp what was happening around and within me. Most importantly, I wanted to make the hurt go away. I saw in theory then a location for healing.

It is in that location that we do the work of language, storytelling, witnessing, releasing, emoting, learning, and connection. We give ourselves a place to put the pain so that it does not solely live in our bodies. We also learn new ways of living as well. When I started my Instagram blog and soon to be website "Black Reading to Heal" it was a response to the work of bell hooks, more specifically *Sisters of the Yams:Black Women & Self-Recovery*. Through a simple practice of highlighting passages, poetry, stories, and more I have had hundreds of Black women write to me about how the work was healing them—hundreds of messages about the benefits to their mental and emotional health. It became absolutely clear to me that writing and reading is a healing approach. It is not inherently healing or radical but when we deliberately undertake the word as such it opens a pathway.

The journey of self-recovery is linked to political resistance. When I began my journey in high school I spent so much time dedicated to self-transformation. The books opened up my worldview and I welcomed the new direction my life would take as I started to identify as a feminist. I wrapped myself up in all the love that was possible. I gave language to my deepest pain and confronted everything sitting in my gut. The more I gave myself a voice through writing the less inflammation, digestive issues, and stomach pain I felt. This was a process that took almost five years. When I faced myself I was then able to realize the aspects of my experience that had nothing to do with me. Ultimately, we cannot self-recover our way out of imperialist white-supremacist capitalist patriarchy or anti-blackness. I was able to see that my suffering was not my own responsibility and that I was not the only person suffering. This would set the foundation for my own political resistance for years to come. Black reading to heal is what Dr. Jameta Barlow would call a "feminist critique with a womanist approach" my approach is to help us "draw up the yams" (hooks, 2005) Meaning, I take the research and turn into praxis. I will always be concerned with the everyday life of Black women and I seek an approach that will work for that context as well. This work becomes important to all other practitioners because it creates a pathway to radicalizing education in all our respective fields. For example, using Black Reading to Heal can draw attention to the alarming number of iconic Black women writers who died of cancer can raise awareness, provide lifesaving information, offer a space of emotional release, and most importantly grapple with revolutionary approaches to end the crisis.

In honor of bell hooks, who honored Toni Cade Bambara by calling the support group she created for Black women students "sisters of the yam," (also her book title) hooks defines the "yam" as: *A life sustaining symbol of black kinship and community. Everywhere black women live in the world, we eat yam. It is a symbol of our diasporic connections. Yams provide nourishment for the body as food yet they are also used medicinally– to heal the body.* bell hooks used Bambara's *The Salt Eaters* to create a healing space and political self-help book for Black women. Bambara reminded me that being well is a hard process. hooks used healing groups to turn the words into praxis. She saw clearly the utility of radical love for Black women's health and creating a loving act when she established these groups. It is in her spirit that I undertake the same mission in my own work. I see the reading of these texts from Black women as running into their arms. When describing "recipes of healing" and ways to ease pain, hooks tells a Black woman: *my remedy is long. But the last item on the list says: when you wake up and find yourself living someplace where there is nobody you love and trust, no community, it is time to leave town—to pack up and go. And where you need to go is any place where there are arms that can hold you, that will not let you go.*

I aim for Black Reading to Heal to become the bridge Black women cross to be held in the arms of Black women via literature. So they can understand that reading can become a liberatory practice. So that they see reading and writing as a spiritual and healing modality. And in all these words they are also gifted new ways of thinking, political strategies, feminist critique, and more. *A practice of love.* Taking the language of Black women writers seriously for our health and for communities. And in this practice we continue to pass down our unique ways of knowing, we honor the work of Black women, and we come together in digital and in person spaces. In this beautiful endeavor, Bambara's love became hooks's love, became my love, . . . and *becomes* your love. We conjure up the deepest feelings we have together. We learn that we are not alone in what we feel or what we have lived. We find each other again and again. We can put our pain right back into the text so that we do not have to carry it all alone. We engage in the practice of memory and its inheritance. Black people all around the world message the blog account calling the post nourishing or helpful. Some people have told me that certain passages shifted their thinking and brought them healing. My favorite responses are the ones where people tell me because of what they read, they discovered a new way to take care of themselves. Every movement or revolutionary requires some level of political education. Providing a political education that seeks to help heal readers and push them toward risk-taking/political resistance is my contribution to the causes I care about. And as republicans continue to ban books and deny children the knowledge needed to become autonomous and self-determining people no one can convince me that this blog is not my own political resistance. We will find ways to get the education, healing, and words to our communities no matter what. We always have.

No one has to view Black women's writings as a bible. But, for me, there are some texts and words that just feel like scripture. Reading is an untenable transformative modality and tool. You have to be vulnerable enough to learn new information and let it transform you. This process requires fortitude and is not to be romanticized either. This is painstaking work that you have to let overtake you. "Are you sure, sweetheart, that you want to be well?. . . Just so you're sure, sweetheart, and ready to be healed, cause wholeness is no trifling matter. A lot of weight when you're well" (Toni Cade Bambara, The Salt Eaters).

Reading and writing to be well is also no trifling matter. Bambara speaks to the painstaking work of love, Black women's inner workings, and healing.

REFERENCES

American Psychiatric Association. (2017). *Mental health facts for African Americans.* Retrieved from https://www.psychiatry.org/psychiatrists/cultural-competency/education/african-american-patients

Collins, P. (2000). *Black Feminist thought: Knowledge, consciousness, and the politics of empowerment* (2nd ed.). New York: Routledge.

Hooks, B. (2001). *All about love* (pp. 55–80). Broadway, New York: William Morrow Paperbacks.

Leggatt-Cook, C. (2010). An uncertain balance: Negotiating theory, politics and love in academic writing. *Feminism & Psychology, 21*(3), 393–410.

Lorde, A. (2007). *Sister outsider* (pp. 45–53). New York: Ten Speed Press.

May, V. M. (2009). Writing the Self into Being: Anna Julia Cooper's Textual Politics. *African American Review*, 43(1), 17–34. http://www.jstor.org/stable/27802556

Nash, J. (2013). Practicing love: Black feminism, love-politics, and post-intersectionality. *Meridians, 11*(2), 1–24.

Phillips, L. (Ed.). (2006). *The womanist reader*. New York: Routledge.

Rickford, R. (2016). *We are an African people: Independent education, Black power, and the radical imagination.* Oxford University Press.

Salecl, R., & Zizek, S. (Eds.). (1996). *Gaze and voice as love objects.* Durham: Duke University Press.

Trudy. (2014). *Black womanhood, asexuality and agency*. Retrieved from http://www.gradientlair.com/post/74476431892/black-woman-asexuality-agency

Taylor, K. (2017). *How we get free: Black feminism and the Combahee river collective* (pp. 10–50). Visionaryproject (2008, December 4).

Toni Morrison talks about her motivation for writing. [video file] Retrieved from https://www.youtube.com/watch?v=_8Zgu2hrs2k

Walker, A. (2005). *Anything we love can be saved* (pp. 10–85). London: Phoenix.

Chapter 5

The Stories We Hold

Health Implications of Embodied Narratives of Black Women and Girls from the Ivory Tower

Chinyere Okafor

BLACK WOMEN AS KNOWLEDGE PRODUCERS

Black women have existed and produced knowledge both within and outside the ivory tower for decades. On the ground, working-class Black women have shown up for their communities as "organic intellectuals" (Gramsci, 1971) wielding knowledge of natural medicines, movement activism, and bridging connections across social networks to equip their communities in the fight for liberation (Harris, 2018; Smith et al., 2021). Within institutions, Georgina Rose Simpson became the first Black woman in the United States to receive a Ph.D. from the University of Chicago in 1921 (Witynski, 2021). It is within these spaces, the "dark hole," that they have imagined and created lanes for themselves in an environment that was not meant to host them apart from extracting labor and demanding silence around their exploitation (Collins, 2000).

In Fall of 2018, the National Center for Education Statistics (2020) recorded that Black women, in consolidation with Black men, Hispanic men, and Hispanic women, made up 3% out of all full-time faculty in degree-granting postsecondary institutions, and only 2% of a full-time professorship. Additionally, in 2016 there were 54,904 doctorate recipients and out of that total, only 1,663 were Black women (Female doctorate recipients, by ethnicity, race, and citizenship status: 2006–16, 2017). These statistics show the staggering numerical reality of Black women's presence in these spaces and hint toward larger structural influences and powers that affect their retention and overall experiences as both graduate students and faculty members.

Utilizing interdisciplinary theories rooted in Black feminist thought, decolonial psychology, and queer theory, this chapter will analyze narrations of navigation and resistance, for Black women, trans, and (non-binary) femme graduate students' mental health outcomes in higher education. Following these threads points us toward necessary examinations of the conditions that impact the bodies and subsequent field of research on Black girls' and women's health. Adopting an interdisciplinary approach is an attempt to dismantle the inflexible categories that exist within health research and writing, to bring forth a "mosaic" approach (Evans-Winters, 2019) that is critical within Black feminist qualitative research. In other words, "discipline is empire," (McKittrick, 2020, p. 36) and by crafting work that incorporates multiple ways of knowing, across a variety of fields and mediums, we can obtain more comprehensive health analyses of this marginalized population.

THE VIOLENT HISTORY OF THE U.S. EDUCATIONAL SYSTEM

There exists a long history of violence toward Black women within the U.S. educational system that includes anti-Black racism, which is the "system of beliefs and practices that attack, erode, and limit the humanity of Black people" (Carruthers, 2018, p. 26) as well as misogynoir, the combination of anti-Blackness and misogyny that simultaneously forces Black women into positions of invisibility and hypervisibility (Bailey, 2014; Bailey, 2018). This violence begins as early as K-12, where research shows Black girls represent less than 17% of total female students but make up 31% of girls sent to law enforcement, and 43% of girls that undergo school-related arrests (Smith-Evans et al., 2014). In every state within the United States, Black girls are more than twice as likely to be suspended from school than their white female counterparts (Camera, 2017). Supplementary research exposes educators placing more focus on the behavior and attitude of Black girls rather than their academic development and emotional and social well-being by utilizing subjective labels like "disruptive" or "defiant" to justify their suspension and/or expulsion (Morris, 2016).

SITUATED KNOWLEDGE OF BLACK FEMMES

Black women within the context of the United States inhabit a particular social-political position as racially gendered subjects. Early Black feminist works sought to explicate the oppressive structures at play in Black women's life experiences. Dr. Patricia Hill Collins speaks about three interdependent dimensions of American Black women's oppression in *Black Feminist Thought* (2000): exploitation of Black women's labor, political subordination, and controlling images. Dr. Kimberlé Crenshaw contributes to this work through her concept of intersectionality (1990), a framework present in early Black feminist writings (Combahee River Collective Statement, 1983) but specifically refers to distinct forms of intersecting oppressions, such as race and gender, that leave Black women vulnerable and virtually invisible in courts of law. Considering these aspects of Black feminist theory, I became enthralled by the ways it emerges within the academy, specifically for Black graduate students who inhabit a more precarious and less powerful position within this institutional structure.

The text *Presumed Incompetent: The Intersections of Race and Class for Women in Academia* (2012) provides countless accounts of the hurdles women faculty of color must navigate within the university system as "marked" bodies and minds. White logic places Black women within a continual position of defeminization that contrasts with the image of the "innocent and domesticated" white woman or white girl (Hines-Datiri & Carter Andrews, 2017). They constantly battle projected ideas of their selfhood, motives, and identity in not only administrative spaces but classrooms as well. Katherine McKittrick states "Learning and teaching and classrooms are, already, sites of pain" (p. 284, 2014). Dehumanizing policies, practices, and interactions with university staff, faculty, and non-Black students greatly impact the safety and well-being of Black women faculty in academic spaces. While there exists a wealth of writing and research on the impact academic institutional violence has on Black women faculty, gaps exist in the health outcomes of Black women, trans, and femme graduate students. Below, I hope to expand my analysis in an attempt to examine this violence against graduate students which is critical for an investigation of the university's problematic structure that allows for violations against the body, mind, and soul of Black women and femme students.

RACISM AND BLACK EMBODIMENT

Racism has long been tracked in health research to have detrimental effects on the psychological and physical health of Black people (Clark et al., 1999). There are a variety of meta-analyses that dive into the negative consequences that these stressors have on the body and mind of Black folk (Pascoe & Richman, 2009). Racism involves both overt and covert acts of violence that at times can operate on more unconscious levels by perpetrators (Lewis et al., 2013). Initially coined by Chester Pierce (1977), a Black psychiatrist, *racial microaggressions* were to help shine a light on the subtle but just as violent racial "slights" that Black people in the United States undergo daily. Contemporary research on microaggressions offers us an in-depth view of the longer-lasting impacts of said violence, indicating negative mental health outcomes like depression for victims (Mazzula & Nadal, 2015). Lewis, Mendenhall, Harwood, and Browne Huntt (2016) illustrate in their work that *gendered racial microaggressions* against Black women emerge in a myriad of ways including but not limited to being treated as a stereotype, experiencing silencing and targeting in workplaces and schools, and negative assumptions made about Black women's body, aesthetic, and intellect (Moody & Lewis, 2019). Overall, research indicates that gendered racial microaggressions are significantly associated with traumatic stress symptoms and responses for Black women (Moody & Lewis, 2019). The scholars call for more research exploring Black women's experiences of discrimination utilizing an intersectional framework as it is one that adequately holds the many revolving pieces of Black woman identity within American society without flattening or reducing the impact that race and gender have on their lives.

When considering the impact of the university on Black women, trans, and femme graduate students bodies, it is important to root ourselves in the current climate of academia in the United States. Though the lasting effects of microaggressions have been made clear, overt violence not only exists within these spaces, but they have also increased over time. The Anti-Defamation League Center on Extremism (COE) (2023) reports that in 2022, there was a significant increase in white supremacist propaganda which includes "the distribution of racist, antisemitic and anti-LGBTQ+ fliers, stickers, banners, graffiti, and posters, as well as laser projections." Their data shows the highest number of propaganda incidents ever recorded, a 38% increase from the previous year (ADL Center on Extremism, 2023). One major site of distribution is college or university campuses which were recorded to have occurred across 39 different states (ADL Center on Extremism, 2023). With this increase of extreme right-wing fascism, the already grim situation for the mental and physical effects on Black women, trans, and femme students does not look bright. Coupled with massive policy changes within the educational system such as the Supreme Court stripping affirmative action from university admissions processes (Totenberg, 2023), alongside an increase in hate crimes in which "race and sexual orientation were the two largest categories of motivating bias associated with the three most common types of hate crimes reported in 2019—intimidation, vandalism, and simple assault" (National Center for Education Statistics, 2022), it is valid to consider the possible lasting effects on these students' educational experience. This is just one snapshot of the campus environment Black women, femme, and trans students are most likely navigating individually and also together. If they are not interacting directly with White nationalist students as classmates, many

Black graduate students interact with them as adjunct professors through yearly teaching fellowships.

PHILOSOPHY OF SCIENCE

Based on the reported statistics and news of increased violence against marginalized people on campus, one can infer how difficult it may be to navigate university spaces as Black women, trans, and femme persons. But what lurks more insidiously beneath these overt displays of hatred are the continuous colonial whispers that bury themselves deep into knowledge production itself. In Linda Tuhiwai Smith's *Decolonizing Methodologies: Research and Indigenous Peoples*, she states, "the term 'research' is inextricably linked to European imperialism and colonialism" (p. 1). Smith peels off the many layers that encapsulate the history of academia to expose its imperial and colonial practices that are shrouded under an academic's pursuit of knowledge. By detailing the ways the West uses research as an imperial technology to "desire, extract and claim ownership of our ways of knowing, our imagery, the things we create and produce, and then simultaneously reject the people who created and developed those ideas and seek to deny them further opportunities to be creators of their own culture and own nations" (p.1), Smith lays out the problems and limitations of this kind of work. She illustrates to her readers that despite good intentions by researchers, academics, and project workers, the belief in the idea that most scientific work is done for the benefit of mankind is still grossly tied to our academic training that remains rooted in colonial and imperial viewpoints. Coming to terms with the inherent nature of research and its history is important for all researchers if the goal is to produce radical and revolutionary work on Black girls' and women's health.

There are a myriad of ways colonial power can be reinscribed within knowledge production, one I'd like to raise is of citational practices. Best described by Ahmed (2014, p. 5),

> Citationality is another form of academic relationality. White men is reproduced as a citational relational. White men cite other white men: it is what they have always done; it is what they will do; what they teach each other to do when they teach each other. They cite; how bright he is; what a big theory he has. He's the next such-and-such male philosopher: don't you think; see him think. The relation is often paternal: the father brings up the son who will eventually take his place. Patriarchy: it's quite a system. It works.

Due to the canon in most academic disciplines grounding themselves in Western, white, male voices, the absence of citing Black women, trans, and femme scholars results in the erasure of their labor, bodies, and mind within intellectual production (Nash, 2020). Scholars (Smith et al., 2021) have traced the historical lineage and parallels between the erasure of Black women's contributions to larger discourses in research, as well as the exploitation, abuse, and misuse of Black women's intellectual property in academic spaces. Cite Black Women (Smith et al., 2021) is just one example of the efforts by Black women to uplift and reinscribe themselves into a history white supremacy fights to hoard space from. As an interdisciplinary collective that includes queer, femme, and gender non-conforming people spanning from a range of disciplines, we are reminded that there is hope; that this work will push for the restructuring and decolonization of the academic structures that exist to harm, undermine, and remove Black women's and femme scholars' outstanding contributions in the pursuit of greater knowledge.

Black femmes are critical to the exploration of their navigation through the colonial neoliberal university. Femme, in this philosophy, is defined as "an inherently queer and political identity that in its essence challenges gender binaries/norms and decenters colonial masculinity to center a more radical, revolutionary gender politic" (Clark, 2019). Their inclusion is important to our examination because there is a particular type of violence inflicted on the bodies of non-men who do not center traditional, western patriarchal notions of masculinity. To leave them out of this conversation is to reify the same power dynamics that the university exalts — dichotomous and hierarchical classifications of humans to further colonial campaigns of dividing and conquering marginalized populations (Lugones, 2010; Yoong & Perkins, 2020).

This erasure also seeps into the important realm of knowledge production and the refusal to examine the structures that also impact Black trans women, femmes, and non-binary femmes becomes another form of epistemic violence (Teo, 2010). Teo (2010) invites us to critically analyze the problem of social-scientific data on the "Other" or marginalized individuals/communities by introducing the concept of epistemological violence within the context of social science research. This violence emerges as the theoretical interpretations of a marginalized group are framed as knowledge rather than interpretations of the data, and said knowledge harms the individual or group due to "misrepresentations and distortions to a neglect of the voices of the 'Other,' to propositions of inferiority, and to the recommendations of adverse practices or infringements concerning the 'Other'" (Teo, 2010). In short, empirical research analyzing Black women, femmes, gender non-conforming, and trans students is at high risk of locating issues of the university against the students rather than the larger processes at work against them due to their social positioning. By constructing Black femmes as 'other' (Spivak, 1988) outside of Black cis women, we ignore the major similarities that overlap across groups that cannot be overlooked, particularly when freedom is on the line.

LOOKING THROUGH BLACK QUEER FEMINIST LENS

Placing attention on Black femmes, gender non-conforming, and trans students' experiences helps us indicate major themes that impact the health of this population as they navigate graduate school. Research indicates trans and non-binary students desiring equality in the school place report that it,

> often fell to individual trans students and staff at significant personal cost; allied to the emotional labour (Hochschild, 2003; Taylor, 2013), time investment and 'outness' this necessitated. Meanwhile, individual practitioners and academics often lacked workload capacity and/or the knowledge, confidence, and intra- and inter-institutional connections to engage in meaningful actions to tangibly advance trans equalities. (Mckendry & Lawrence, 2020)

Over the last few years, particularly during the Trump administration, governmental departments and agencies such as the Department of Education, the Department of Justice, and the Health and Human Services Office for Civil Rights have undone a variety of safeguards for the LGBTQIA+ community (Shelton & Lester, 2022). Healthcare disparities within this community are directly and intimately tied to the sexual and social stigma that has stalked them for decades (Lim, Brown Jr, & Kim, 2014). As a result, an already vulnerable population of our society has witnessed and faced the destruction of protections in the arenas of healthcare, housing, and education (Lovelace, 2019; Shelton & Lester, 2022).

Despite these changes affecting the broader queer community, Black trans and non-binary people are immoderately burdened by these changes, with Black trans women and femmes in particular who risk higher rates of murder due to transphobia and racism (Shelton & Lester, 2022; GLAAD, 2019; Carpenter & Marshall, 2017). Julia Serano (2007) coined the concept *transmisogyny* which describes and argues that trans women face a particular oppression due to the devaluation of femininity alongside transgenderism. However, many scholars argue that due to the concept centering on the lives of mostly white, middle-class trans women, as well as Serano's use of rigid definitions and binaries of trans identity and presentation, there are limits to its efficacy in describing the fullness of Black trans experience, particularly when the categories constructed do not honor the violence Black and native bodies have been subjected to from the medical industry (Krell, 2017). As a result, adopting the term *transmisogynoir* highlights the ways racism, anti-Blackness, and transmisogyny combine to impact the lives of Black trans women and femmes (Stewart & Nicolazzo, 2018). Understanding the terms and theories surrounding the interlocking systems of oppression for Black trans people assists in elucidating the institutionalized obstacles and barriers that impact both their health and access to healthcare. In doing so, researchers conducting work with this population can avoid limited and problematic discussions on Black trans people and health by refusing to make large, generalized discussions of the trans community that currently exists in most quantitative health research (Shelton & Lester, 2022; Buge et al., 2016).

Following this inclusion of Black trans women's and femmes' experience within higher education, la paperson (2017) offers a useful description of the movement of Black femmes in the context of cinema that can translate into their movement within the academic environment,

> The Black Femme is violently pushed aside in commonsense notions of radical Black politics . . .. the Black Femme is there, appearing and then disappearing to the offscreen world. Just beyond the frame, she is a "seething spectral presence" that disrupts the common sense of hegemonic Black masculinity and attendant forms of Black womanhood that have become the metonyms for Black radical politics and revolutionary change. In this respect, the Black Femme is a spectral figure, who when followed, leads us to "a more radical elsewhere"—a world just beyond the frame, with imaginaries of justice and gender and ways of being-in-community that are alternatives from the cinematic common sense.

This spectral figure deserves to be engaged. She leads us to these liberatory spaces of freedom and new ways of being that cannot be ignored within our understanding of Black health. Because the Black woman and the Black femme guide us to emancipatory places imaginatively and materially, recentering them together in the frame of this work directs us not only to deeper understandings of the racist, classist, sexist, and queerphobic threads that keep the neoliberal university afloat, but also to places of joy, dreaming, healing, and care that were never a part of the university in the first place.

McKittrick (2020, p. 27) reminds us that there have always been "Black ways of knowing and living" that have involved overturning the knowledge systems upheld in institutional scholarship. In embracing Black feminist consciousness in our approach to research and analysis on the health of Black girls, women, trans, and femme people, I am led to the work of Dr. Venus Evans-Winters (2019) who states that adopting this lens shapes "(1) musings about knowledge and knowing, (2) how one interacts wih participants throughout the research process, (3) one's understanding of the context where the study takes place, (4) the body of literature reviewed, and (5) interpretation and analysis of data." Such an orientation drastically changes traditional notions and approaches to public health research. Including Black femmes in my analysis is a response to Muñoz's (2006) call to "imagine a position or narrative of being and becoming that can resist the pull of identarian models of relationality" and lean into the forgotten histories and political traditions of Black feminist theory that is not just a synonym to intersectionality, but one that radically invests in both similarity and difference as a project and commitment of love (Nash, 2011).

THE SETTLER COLONIAL PROJECT AND VIOLENCE OF THE UNIVERSITY

Black femme and non-binary students in the classroom experience threats to their emotional safety through microaggressions such as misgendering by both faculty and students, which at times results in many remaining closeted out and/or altering their appearance out of fear (Goldberg & Kuvalanka, 2019). Trans college students have also reported greater exposure to harassment and discrimination on campus, and a lower sense of belonging, compared to cisgender students (Garvey & Rankin, 2015; Rankin & Beemyn, 2012). Black trans women and femmes have been arrested on graduate school campuses on charges of "manifesting prostitution" (Stewart & Nicolazzo, 2022) for merely walking to class, framed as problems by faculty and staff (Butler, 2004; Spade, 2015), are subject to administrative violence (Spade, 2015), and are relatively ignored when faced with individual biases of their personhood by faculty and students. More research is needed to unpack how race impacts femme and non-binary students in both college and higher education spaces and this chapter attempts to open that door by bringing them into the conversation and pointing us to areas cis-gendered-based work can improve.

Furthermore, to understand the mechanisms at work against this marginalized group of students, we must critically examine the university as a whole. The text, *A Third University is Possible* (paperson, 2017) delineates the many moving parts of the settler colonial project and violence of the university on not only Black, Brown, and Indigenous students, faculty, and workers, but also the land, the communities around it, and the overall future of academic (more specifically third world feminist, Black, and Indigenous) studies and work. The text offers a framework of four worlds to understand the university: the first world university is the academic-industrial complex ("research ones") and commercial universities whose commitment is to brand expansion, publication, and prestige; the second world university comprises independent or "liberal arts" colleges that promote art, humanities, and a "libertarian" mode of critical thinking which displaces the opportunity of sustained, radical critique; the third world university defines itself as an interdisciplinary and transnational decolonial project that equips students with the skills for the applied practice of decolonization (paperson, 2017). Examining the multiple forms that the university functions, it allows space for identifying the university model students are enrolled in as well as the specific issues that they are navigating.

SPIRIT MURDER

A deeper analysis of the university points us to neocolonial threads that interlace and expose a complicated web of plantation politics. Many scholars have written about the parallels between slave plantations and contemporary universities (Tuitt, Squire, & Williams, 2018; Williams, Squire, & Tuitt, 2021). Some works have referred to predominantly white institutions (PWIs) as "slave plantations" (Durant, 1999) which highlights the relationship in which there are "defined roles, social positions, norms, and relationships among slaves and non-slaves within a social hierarchy based on race and class." Utilizing this metaphor, Young and Hines (2018) illustrate how Black women professors experience "spirit-murdering" by white students and faculty which becomes an analogy to the killings of Black women by police. The authors state,

> We attest that black women professors are being spirit-murdered on the plantation of academia to kill their physical body through removal, to murder their minds, and to fatally pierce their souls. The spirit-murdering of black female faculty deserts them into a spiritual dying where they will ultimately not have the strength and ethos to unchain themselves. (p. 20)

Young and Hines (2018) offer up three forms of spirit murders by white students at PWIs: (1) personal attacks and deflecting, (2) denigration of course content, and (3) presumed pedagogical incompetence (p. 20). What is significant about these findings is that Black femme and women graduate students are not exempt from experiencing these forms of spirit murders, particularly from white students and faculty within and outside of their department. This becomes key in identifying the structures in place and the mechanisms of violence that plague a community of people even more ignored based on their positionality in the hierarchy of the academic totem pole. This segues into examining the institutional violence Black women and femmes experience as students in higher education.

PEDAGOGIES OF SURVIVAL

Glover (2017) offers critical, personal, and valuable insight into the world of navigating and surviving academia as a Black lesbian graduate student. She raises the question, "Who will fight for our lives but us?".The question Glover encourages us to investigate also illustrates that part of this survival involves leaning into other Black women and femme students or faculty for support, affirmation, guidance, and help due to the failure of the university. As Cahill (2021) similarly expresses,

> Most of my life I have pursued academics and organizing in service of Blackgirls. I have often felt like an outsider: too feminist, too Black, too introverted, and/or too overwhelmed in the politics of care and process over direct action. But in spite of those feelings of lack, I always feel most seen, loved, and held by other Blackgirls. The ritualized work and service they offer to me, their families, their community, and the world are unparalleled. The collective struggle Blackgirls have engaged in to (re)imagine and create a society more free, more equitable, and more magical—is love of a radical form. (Moore, 2018)

Cahill identifies the anguish involved in inhabiting these spaces and that due to this shared struggle, other Black girls' support aids in mitigating the harm. Glover's piece helps give texture and firsthand accounts of the matrix/whirlpool of violence that one must combat daily in academia. She highlights the trauma of being positioned as the problem for "talking back" against gendered racist situations by both instructors and peers (p. 157), the dehumanization of tokenism (p. 162), the policing of affects (p. 162), advising fiascos, and the rude awakening of undergoing this treatment in a program slated as feminist and social justice oriented.

THE POWER OF STORYTELLING AND COUNTERNARRATIVES

Storytelling and examining narratives allow one to make sense of our environment, experiences, and the meaning of the world (Chase, 2003). By engaging with personal stories, we can draw from a wealth of information that highlights not only the tale being told but also the contradictions and nuances that can emerge from its share (Okafor, 2018). Canham and Langa (2017) state that "narrative methods which elicit stories are able to tap into this despair. But they do more. They enable a complexity which is closer to the realities of everyday life." Unfortunately, there exists a long history of scientific racism in research like psychology and other health disciplines that construct damage-centered narratives of racialized groups (Teo, 2011; Tuck, 2009). By dethroning white, Western accounts of Black women and femmes, we begin to engage in the process of decolonization where storytelling from the eye of the oppressed challenges dominant colonial perspectives (Samuel & Ortiz, 2021; Adams et al., 2015). Individual narratives can challenge long-held beliefs and judgments, particularly the accounts that emerge from the life stories of people who are historically silenced (Balaram, 2021). The following sections will explore narrations by Black women and femme graduate students to gain deeper insight into the connection between academic violence and health outcomes.

bell hooks, in "Talking Back: Thinking Feminist, Thinking Black" (2014), writes about her experiences as a graduate student where she witnessed a myriad of racist and sexist humiliations and terrorization aimed at students to shame and break their spirit.. She discusses the process of navigating the space by avoiding classes taught by racist professors or the difficulty of finding a professor that would take the accusations seriously. Changing hiring practices meant an increase of Black professors, but their presence can only mediate white violence in a minor way due to the plight of Black faculty in universities who must hold the large labor of their position, teaching duties, and mentoring students of color. The following quote centers on her experience of racism and sexism with a white male professor of American literature,

> He was telling me that I could avoid the systematic abuse by simply dropping out. I would not drop out. I continued to work even though it was clear that I would not succeed, even as the persecution became more intense. And even though I constantly resisted. In time, my spirits were more and more depressed. I began to dream of entering the professor's office with a loaded gun. There I would demand that he listen, that he experience the fear, the humiliation. In my dreams I could hear his pleading voice begging me not to shoot, to remain calm. As soon as I put the gun down he would become his old self again. Ultimately in the dream the only answer was to shoot, to shoot to kill. When this dream became so consistently a part of my waking fantasies, I knew that it was time for me to take a break from graduate school. (p. 58)

hooks' account illustrates the lasting impact on her mental, emotional, and physical health due to enduring racial-gendered abuse. Its pervasiveness led to visions of her enacting the same violence that she suffered against her harm-doer, something out of character and against the values that she held. What is also significant to note in her account is the eventual "pushout" (Morris, 2016) that led her to leave the graduate school space to preserve and tend to her health.

In Michele Wallace's critical text "Invisibility Blues" (1990) she discusses not only her own experience navigating graduate school but also draws upon its generational ties to the experience of her aunt who also attempted to receive a terminal degree. In a snippet detailing her own story she writes,

> In the search for validation, I landed in the Phd program in American Studies at Yale, where I was lost before I started. . . . While I could write reasonably well, and I read a lot, the words seemed to escape me when it was time to talk to fellow graduate students. I was morbidly afraid that when I opened my mouth, I would show my bottomless ignorance and make a fool of myself. So I kept to myself and read voraciously but came to loathe the superbly well-educated, articulate whites who shared my classes. I feared I would never catch up. When

> the fear became too much for me — I was no brave person either — I dropped out. But the project of catching up will always describe my existential plight. (p. 97)

Wallace illustrates the isolation and fear inherent in inhabiting a white academic institutional space as a Black woman, particularly during a time when Black women and femmes were less present and admitted in higher education programs than in our contemporary time. The fear became so all-consuming that it also eventually led to her exit from the program with little to no discussion on how the program, its faculty, or the larger school offered resources, support, or even care toward her absence. When discussing the story of her Aunt Barbara she shares,

> I don't know precisely when she completed her master's, but remember her briefly pursuing her PhD at Columbia, then dropping out because a professor accused her of being illiterate, although I always thought she spoke the most precise English and read more books than anybody I ever knew. . . . As an elementary school teacher, she grew to hate the public schools. About five years ago she drank herself to death. (p. 96)

Analyzing this quote allows us access to a rare vantage point that acknowledges a generational pattern rooted in structural violence against a specific marginalized group. The failures present in multiple levels of educational spaces potentially contributed to the physical damage and emotional turmoil within Aunt Barbara's body and untimely death. Experiencing racism in one's daily life means one is in a continuous condition of danger, becoming a social exposure that increases levels of cortisol due to stress and making one susceptible to developing disorders and diseases (Barlow & Johnson, 2021). These accounts illustrate that these abuses are to not be taken lightly when lives are sequentially threatened by this violence.

In a return to Glover's story, she names the following factors that challenged her belonging, safety, and wellness in graduate school spaces: regional racial and sexual politics; misogynoir and homophobia; myths of safety and community; asymmetrical solidarity; professionalization cultures; and "pedagogy of accommodation" (p. 158). The significance of this piece is not only the detailed examinations of her position as a queer Black woman within academia but also the insight she offers into the lasting effects both mentally and physically on her body. This indicates the violence and spirit murders that occur against the bodies of Black women and femme graduate students that very easily evolve into physical ailments. Glover shares,

> While in my master's program, at the tender age of twenty-two, I began to suffer from debilitating chronic neck, shoulder, and back pain, which I learned from

> doctors was because of subluxations, or misaligned vertebrae, and a deteriorating spinal disk that correlated to constant poor posture from extended laptop use and reading, as well as carrying heavy books. . . . Most importantly, subluxations can occur at any age, and the main causes are considered the "Three Ts": trauma, toxins, and thoughts—with thoughts/stress being the number one cause, followed by both micro and major trauma. . . . Essentially, this world and this environment was killing me slowly—constantly experiencing racialized and homophobic familial crises, financial crises, microaggressions and lack of safety, being tense and criminalized all of the time in the white and respectable environments, being disconnected from cultural expression central to my life force and catharsis, having no time to maintain wellness rituals, relationships, or get enough rest due to the large workload and its demands. The stress, trauma, and distrust I felt for white people during my first PWI experience became compounded by the incessant Black deaths from police brutality reported in the media. Plus, given my research and subjectivity, the sociopolitical moment underlined how anti-Black violence against Black cis and transwomen fails to galvanize the same mourning and fervor for redress. I suffered from muscle spasms and inability to sleep comfortably because of muscle tension; and I developed anxiety and panic attacks for the first time in my life. (p. 170)

Glover offers us an in-depth analysis of the relationship between her health decline to her presence of existing and navigating academic violence as a Black femme graduate student. The disturbing truth is how interrelated it is to stories of well-known academics like Audre Lorde and June Jordan who, in a piece shared by Alexis Pauline Gumbs (2012), had deaths directly related to the denial of medical leave by their universities after being diagnosed with cancer. In other words, the health of Black women and femme graduate students and faculty are impacted by both direct and indirect violence implemented within the infrastructure of the university system.

DECOLONIZATION AND HEALING WITHIN HEALTH SCIENCES

Though this is not the case for all graduate school experiences, isolation and loneliness remain for many current Black women and femme graduate students, especially during our current reality of COVID. It is important and healing to write about our experiences and more specifically, survival strategies. There is immense power in developing critical consciousness to thoughtfully reflect on your lived experience, analyze your sociopolitical climate, and determine what steps of action are available for one to create change (Mosley et al., 2020). By building said consciousness and exploring it through writing, Black girls and women can promote healing individually and collectively. Education is not a neutral process. Richard Shaull (1991) states in his introduction to Freire's *Pedagogy of the Oppressed*,

> Education either functions as an instrument which is used to facilitate the integration of the younger generation into the logic of the present system and bring about conformity to it, or it becomes the "practice of freedom", the means by which men and women deal critically and creatively with reality and discover how to participate in the transformation of the world

To decolonize the university, we must see it as an active practice that not only reaches us cognitively as a metaphor, but also on a structural, affective, embodied, and soul level (Tuck & Yang, 2012). As a larger epistemological approach to Black girls, women, and femmes' health, decolonization becomes a drastic but necessary process to produce accurate research that addresses all the interlocking systems of oppression that work to minimize, devalue, and dehumanize this population in both method and theoretical grounding. In a piece titled "Beyond the Side Eye: Black Women's Ancestral Anger as a Liberatory Practice" (2017) by Dr. Julia S. Jordan-Zachery, she investigates anger as a haunting from generations of Black women that brings forth political action. Black Feminist Hauntology is defined as "an anti-colonial analysis of time that captures the expanding and repetitive nature of structural violence, a process whereby we begin to locate a language to speak about the actual, not just symbolic or theorized violence that is racial colonialism" (p. 62).

Embracing this haunting while holding these narratives as qualitative truth helps us explore the lived experiences, traumas, and emotions of Black women and femmes within the academy. By examining these narratives, we can begin to identify the intricate strands holding these stories of academic abuse to the subsequent health challenges experienced by this marginalized group. In centering the everydayness of this violence and how its hauntings affect mental health, physical health, and healing for this population, we as researchers can shift our focus to these private spheres that many health researchers would rather ignore. Engaging hauntings as a methodological approach in health research means to recenter their voices in an effort to highlight the external oppressive structures in place within the academy that typically go unnamed.

Emphasizing these stories that are embedded in the bodies of Black women and femme graduate students can point us toward pathways of healing and support that they need. Their positionality highlights particular structural issues that in addressing can mitigate further mental harm for future generations of not only this population of students but ALL students. Decolonization is essential and academic programs need more than just superficial diversity, equity, and inclusion offices but a complete overhaul of the colonial vestiges that continue to wreak havoc on Black marginalized gendered bodies. Through these hauntings, we are pointed toward resources and systems of change to improve both the mental and physical health of graduate students everywhere. By embracing not only these stories of harm but ones of care, love, hope, and joy for this community, we will be able to imagine new constructions of these spaces for the healthy continuation of scholars everywhere.

REFERENCES

Adams, G., Dobles, I., Gomez, L. H., Kurtis, T., & Molina, L. E. (2015). Decolonizing psychological science: Introduction to the special thematic section. *Journal of Social and Political Psychology, 3*(1), 213–238. https://doi.org/10.23668/psycharchives.1766

ADL Center on Extremism. (2023, March 8). *White supremacist propaganda soars to all-time high in 2022*. ADL. https://www.adl.org/resources/report/white-supremacist-propaganda-soars-all-time-high-2022

Ahmed, S. (2014). White men. *Feminist Killjoys*, 4.

Bailey, M. (2014, April 27). More on the origins of misogynoir. Moyazb. http://moyazb. tumblr.com/post/84048113369/more-on-the-origin-of-misogynoir

Bailey, M., & Trudy. (2018). On misogynoir: Citation, erasure, and plagiarism. *Feminist Media Studies, 18*(4), 762–768.

Balaram, A. (2021). Crafting new narratives of diasporic resistance with Indo-Caribbean women and gender-expansive people across generations. *Societies, 11*(1), 2.

Barlow, J. N., & Johnson, B. M. (2021). Listen to black women: Do black feminist and womanist health policy analyses. *Women's Health Issues, 31*(2), 91–95.

Budge, S. L., Thai, J. L., Tebbe, E. A., & Howard, K. A. S. (2016). The intersection of race, sexual orientation, socioeconomic status, trans identity, and mental health outcomes. *Counseling Psychologist, 44*, 1025–1049.

Butler, J. (2004). *Undoing gender*. Psychology Press.

Cahill, L. (2021). Radical love unlimited: A biomythography. *Visual Arts Research, 47*(1), 89–100.

Canham, H., & Langa, M. (2017). Narratives of everyday resistance from the margins. *Psychology in Society, 55*, 3–13.

Camera, L. (2017, May 9). *Black girls are twice as likely to be suspended, in every state*. U.S. News & World Report. https://www.usnews.com/news/education-news/articles/2017-05-09/black-girls-are-twice-as-likely-to-be-suspended-in-every-state

Campt, T. M. (2019, December). *The loophole of retreat-an invitation*. https://www.e-flux.com/journal/105/302556/the-loophole-of-retreat-an-invitation/

Carpenter, L. F., & Marshall, R. B. (2017). Walking while trans: Profiling of transgender women by law enforcement, and the problem of proof. *William & Mary Journal of Race, Gender, and Social Justice, 24*(1), 1–35.

Carruthers, C. (2018). *Unapologetic: A black, queer, and feminist mandate for radical movements*. Boston, MA: Beacon Press.

Chase, S. E. (2003). Learning to listen: Narrative principles in a qualitative research methods course. In R. Josselson, A. Lieblich, & D. P. McAdams (Eds.), *Up close and personal: The teaching and learning of narrative research* (pp. 79–99). American Psychological Association. https://doi.org/10.1037/10486-005e.

Clark, R. personal communication/interview, October 8, 2019.

Clark, R., Anderson, N. B., Clark, V. R., & Williams, D. R. (1999). Racism as a stressor for African Americans: A biopsychosocial model. *American Psychologist*, *54*(10), 805.

Collective, C. R. (1983). The Combahee river collective statement, April 1977. *Home Girls: A Black Feminist Anthology*, 272–282.

Collins, P. H. (2000). *Black feminist thought: Knowledge, consciousness, and the politics of empowerment*. New York: Routledge.

Crenshaw, K. (1990). Mapping the margins: Intersectionality, identity politics, and violence against women of color. *Stanford Law Review*, *43*, 1241.

Durant Jr, T. J. (1999). The slave plantation revisited: A sociological perspective. In Thomas J. Durant & J. David Knottnerus (Ed.), *Plantation society and race relations: The origins of inequality* (pp. 3–15). London: Bloomsbury Publishing.

Evans-Winters, V. E. (2019). *Black feminism in qualitative inquiry: A mosaic for writing our daughter's body*. Routledge.

Garvey, J. C., & Rankin, S. R. (2015). The influence of campus experiences on the level of outness among trans-spectrum and queer-spectrum students. *Journal of Homosexuality*, 62, 374–393. http://doi.org/10.1080/00918369.2014.977113

Giddings, P. (1984). *When and where I enter: The impact of Black women on race and sex in America*. New York: Bantam.

GLAAD. (2019, October). GLAAD calls for increased and accurate media coverage of transgender murders. https://www.glaad.org/blog/glaad-calls-increased-and-accurate-media-coverage-transgender-murders-0

Gramsci, A. (1971). *Selections from the prison notebooks of Antonio Gramsci*. New York: International Publishers.

Glover, S. T. (2017). "Black Lesbians—Who will fight for our lives but Us?": Navigating power, belonging, labor, resistance, and graduate student survival in the Ivory tower. *Feminist Teacher*, *27*(2–3), 157–175.

Goldberg, A. E., & Kuvalanka, K. (2019). Transgender graduate students' experiences in higher education: A mixed-methods exploratory study. *Journal of Diversity in Higher Education*, *12*(1), 38.

Gutiérrez y Muhs, G., Niemann, Y. F., González, C. G., & Harris, A. P. (2012). Presumed incompetent: The intersections of race and class for women in academia.

Gumbs, A. P. (2012). The shape of my impact. *The Feminist Wire*, *29*(1). http://thefeministwire.com/2012/10/theshapeofmyimpact/

Harris, C. (2018). The Black organic intellectual tradition and the challenges of educating and developing organic intellectuals in the 21st century. *Journal of Intersectionality*, *2*(1), 51–107.

Hines-Datiri, D., & Carter Andrews. The effects of zero-tolerance policies on Black girls: Using critical race feminism and figured worlds to examine school discipline. Urban Education, published online February 15, 2017. https://doi.org/0042085917690204

Hudson, P. J., & McKittrick, K. (2014). The geographies of blackness and anti-blackness: An interview with Katherine McKittrick. *The CLR James Journal, 20*(1/2), 233–240.

Hooks, B. (1989). *Talking back: Thinking feminist, thinking black* (Vol. 10). South End Press.

Jordan-Zachery, J. S. (2017). Beyond the side eye: Black women's ancestral anger as a liberatory practice. *Journal of Black Sexuality and Relationships*, *4*(1), 61–81.

Krell, E. C. (2017). Is transmisogyny killing trans women of color? Black trans feminisms and the exigencies of white femininity. *Transgender Studies Quarterly*, *4*(2), 226–242.

Lewis, J. A., Mendenhall, R., Harwood, S. A., & Browne Huntt, M. (2013). Coping with gendered racial microaggressions among Black women college students. *Journal of African American Studies*, *17*, 51–73.

Lewis, J. A., Mendenhall, R., Harwood, S., & Browne Huntt, M. (2016). "Ain't I a woman?": Perceived genderedracial microaggressions experienced by Black women. *The Counseling Psychologist*, *44*, 758–780. https://doi.org/10.1177/0011000016641193

Lovelace, B. (2019, May). Trump administration to roll-back health care protections for transgender people. CNBC. https://www.cnbc.com/2019/05/24/trump-administration-to-roll-back-health-protections-for-transgender.html

Lugones, M. (2010). Toward a decolonial feminism. *Hypatia*, *25*(4), 742–759.

Mazzula, S. L., & Nadal, K. L. (2015). Racial microaggressions, whiteness, and feminist therapy. *Women & Therapy*, *38*(3–4), 308–326.

McKittrick, K. (2020). *Dear science and other stories*. Duke University Press.

Moody, A. T., & Lewis, J. A. (2019). Gendered racial microaggressions and traumatic stress symptoms among Black women. *Psychology of Women Quarterly*, *43*(2), 201–214.

Morris, M. (2016). *Pushout: The criminalization of Black girls in schools*. New Press.

Mosley, D. V., Hargons, C. N., Meiller, C., Angyal, B., Wheeler, P., Davis, C., & Stevens-Watkins, D. (2021). Critical consciousness of anti-Black racism: A practical model to prevent and resist racial trauma. *Journal of Counseling Psychology*, *68*(1), 1–16. https://doi.org/10.1037/cou0000430

Muñoz, J. (2006). Feeling brown, feeling down: Latina affect, the performativity of race, and the depressive position. *Signs*, *31*(3), 675–88.

Nash, J. C. (2013). Practicing love: Black feminism, love-politics, and post-intersectionality. *Meridians, 11*(2), 1–24.

Nash, J. C. (2020). Citational Desires: On Black Feminism's Institutional Longings. *Diacritics*, *48*(3), 76–91.

National Center for Education Statistics. (2022). Hate crime incidents at postsecondary institutions. *Condition of Education*. U.S. Department of Education, Institute of Education Sciences. Retrieved June 27, 2023, from https://nces.ed.gov/programs/coe/indicator/a22

Okafor, C. (2018). Black feminism embodiment: A theoretical geography of home, healing, and activism. *Meridians*, *16*(2), 373–381.

paperson, la. (2017). *A third university is possible*. University of Minnesota Press.

Pascoe, E. A., & Smart Richman, L. (2009). Perceived discrimination and health: a meta-analytic review. *Psychological Bulletin, 135*(4), 531.
Pierce, C. M., Carew, J. V., Pierce-Gonzalez, D., & Wills, D. (1977). An experiment in racism: TV commercials. *Education and Urban Society, 10*, 61–87.
Rankin, S., & Beemyn, G. (2012). Beyond a binary: The lives of gender nonconforming youth. *About Campus: Enriching the Student Learning Experience, 17*, 2–10. http://doi.org/10.1002/abc.21086
Samuel, C. A., & Ortiz, D. L. (2021). "Method and meaning": Storytelling as decolonial praxis in the psychology of racialized peoples. *New Ideas in Psychology, 62*, 100868.
Shaull, R. (1991). *The reformation and liberation theology: Insights for the challenges of today*. Westminster John Knox Press.
Serano, J. (2007). *Whipping girl: A transsexual woman on sexism and the scapegoating of femininity*. Emeryville, CA: Seal.
Shelton, S. A., & Lester, A. O. (2022). A narrative exploration of the importance of intersectionality in a Black trans woman's mental health experiences. *International Journal of Transgender Health, 23*(1–2), 108–121.
Smith, L. T. (2021). *Decolonizing methodologies: Research and indigenous peoples*. Bloomsbury Publishing.
Smith, C. A., Williams, E. L., Wadud, I. A., Pirtle, W. N., & Cite Black Women Collective. (2021). Cite black women: A critical praxis (a statement). *Feminist Anthropology, 2*(1), 10–17.
Smith-Evans, L., George, J., Graves, F., Kaufmann, L., & Frohlich, L. (2014). Unlocking opportunity for African American girls. Retrieved from https://nwlc.org/wp-content/uploads/2015/08/unlocking_opportunity_for_african_american_girls_report.pdf.
Spade, D. (2015). *Normal life: Administrative violence, critical trans politics, and the limits of law*. Durham, NC: Duke University Press.
Spivak, G. C. (1988). Can the subaltern speak? In C. Nelson & L. Grossberg (Eds.), *Marxism and the interpretation of culture* (pp. 271–313). Urbana: University of Illinois Press.
Stewart, D. L., & Nicolazzo, Z. (2018). High impact of [whiteness] on trans* students in postsecondary education. *Equity & Excellence in Education, 51*(2), 132–145.
Sue, D. W. (2010). *Microaggressions in everyday life: Race, gender, and sexual orientation*. Hoboken: Wiley & Sons, Inc.
Teo, T. (2010). What is epistemological violence in the empirical social sciences? *Social and Personality Psychology Compass, 4*(5), 295–303.
Totenberg, N. (2023, June 29). *Supreme court guts affirmative action, effectively ending race-conscious admissions*. NPR. https://www.npr.org/2023/06/29/1181138066/affirmative-action-supreme-court-decision
Tuck, E. (2009). Suspending damage: A letter to communities. *Harvard Educational Review, 79*(3), 409–428.
Tuck, E., & Yang, K. W. (2012). Decolonization is not a metaphor. *Decolonization: Indigeneity, Education & Society, 1*(1), 19–22.
Tuitt, F., Squire, D., & Williams, B. (2018). Plantation politics and neoliberal racism in higher education: A framework for reconstructing anti-racist institutions. *Teachers College Record, 120*(14), 1–20.

U.S. Department of Education, National Center for Education Statistics. (2020). *The condition of education 2020* (NCES 2020-144). Characteristics of Postsecondary Faculty.

Wallace, M. (1990). *Invisibility blues: From pop to theory*. Verso.

Williams, B. C., Squire, D. D., & Tuitt, F. A. (Eds.). (2021). *Plantation politics and campus rebellions: Power, diversity, and the emancipatory struggle in higher education*. State University of New York Press.

Witynski, M. (2021, June 10). *100 years ago, Georgiana Simpson made history as the first black woman to graduate with a Ph.D.* University of Chicago News. https://news.uchicago.edu/story/100-years-ago-georgiana-simpson-made-history-first-black-woman-graduate-phd#:~:text=100%20years%20ago%2C%20Georgiana%20Simpson,University%20of%20Chicago%20News

Yoong, D. D., & Perkins, K. M. (2020). Flowing between the personal and collective: Being human beyond categories of study. *Societies*, *10*(4), 94.

Young, J. L., & Hines, D. E. (2018). Killing my spirit, renewing my soul: Black female professors' critical reflections on spirit killings while teaching. *Women, Gender, and Families of Color*, *6*(1), 18–25.

Chapter 6

Welcome to the Kitchen Table

Where Stories and Images Center the Lived Experiences of Black Women and Their Bodies

Y. Falami Devoe

For six weeks, they gathered. They gathered, exchanging
stories and tears . . . memories
and smiles. Exchanging life stories from past to present . . . reflecting on the future.
Sitting around the *virtual "kitchen table," ten women, ten "sisters" not by blood . . .
but shared experiences
came together to
share and unpack
the lived experiences
of their bodies . . .
never before
had any
had
a conversation
like this.
Welcome to the kitchen table.

*Virtual kitchen table—a space likened to kitchen tables in homes within Black communities where individuals are nourished and fed not only food but nourished by conversation and community.

And the sitting at the kitchen table continues; not only kitchen tables, but beauty shops, sister circles, podcasts, online communities, and social media platforms. These places and spaces, brave, free, unapologetically Black, unrestrained Female energy abound are where mothers, "other mothers," "sisters," "sister friends," cousins, and girlfriends connect, listen, bond, affirm, share, and heal in community. Phillips (2006) highlights this kitchen table metaphor for understanding the Womanist perspective on dialogue and the benefits of these spaces:

The "kitchen table" is an informal woman-centered space where all are welcome and all can participate. The table is an invitation to become part of a group amicably comprised of heterogeneous elements and unified by the pleasure and nourishment of food and drink. At the table, people can come and go, agree or disagree, take turns talking or speak all at once, and laugh, should, complain, or counsel—even be present in silence. At the kitchen table, people share the truths of their lives on equal footing and learn through face-to-face conversation. (xxvii)

These communal spaces are Womanist spaces.

PHILOSOPHY OF SCIENCE

My philosophy of science seeks to elucidate the value in and of communal spaces and the collective ways of sharing and processing lived experiences, challenge the process of doing research "with" Black women and girls instead of "on" and center embodiment of Black women and girls and their bodies through the utilization of images and collective conversations around "the kitchen table."

I exist at the intersection of my race, gender, and sexual orientation. Existing at these crossroads provides a lens in which I see and feel not only my experiences with my body present and past but the experiences of Black women's and girls' bodies present. From the age of 4, I was raised by my mother. My mother, a native of the south, reared by two parents, instilled in me Christian values and morals. These Christian values and morals were very much rooted in patriarchy, Eurocentricity, and heteronormativity. These values were seen in the expectations that were communicated verbally and non-verbally around what it meant to be and look like a lady, rooted in Eurocentric ideologies of beauty and behavior. In addition to the Eurocentric ideologies of beauty and behavior that were instilled in me, was the undergird of the Christian Church, which was to control and conform.. As a Black lesbian who came out later in life, I have navigated what W.E.B Dubois calls "Double Consciousness." Dubois (2008) stated "It is a peculiar sensation, this double-consciousness, this sense of always looking at one's self through the eyes of others, of measuring one's soul by the tape of a world that looks on in amused contempt and pity. One ever feels his two-ness, – an American, a Negro; two souls, two thoughts, two unreconciled strivings; two warring ideals in one dark body, whose dogged strength alone keeps it from being torn asunder" (Du Bois, *The Souls of Black Folk*, p. 2).

Yes, Dubois was referring to the angst of living and navigating in a society not meant for Black folks. However, Double Consciousness is applicable to anyone like myself, who is a minoritized member of the LGBTQIA + community and lives under the guise of the heteronormativity. From childhood to adulthood, my life and body have been controlled not only by those closest to me but others who had a marked influence on my life. This control often times left me silent or lacking authenticity. I commit to center and provide space for Black girls and Women to dialogue and enter into a space where they may find healing. I was drawn to Womanism after reading and reflecting on Walker's 1985 definition of Womanism. I was captivated because every essence of that definition was me past and present. When I began my research study, and began to read a plethora of Womanist Scholars, I found the holistic discussion of Womanism by Layli (Phillips) Mayparyan, relevant to my praxis as a Womanist and the theoretical underpinning for my study. Maparyan (2012) elucidates the power of dialogue within the Womanist worldview. "When two or more people engage in dialogue, the power of the word is amplified and energetic gears of influence upon material reality are automatically set into motion" (p. 60). As a Womanist scholar, there is power in dialogue (Maparyan, 2012).

I AM A WOMANIST!

A Womanist is one who boldly searches for deeper meaning and greater truths counter to what is considered good for one. She loves, appreciates, honors, celebrates the beauty, strength, and vulnerability of women. She connects with spirit, mind, and body, and is committed to the survival and wholeness of humanity. Assertion, agency, and acknowledgement are words which thematically undergird Alice Walker's (1985) definition of a Womanist and Womanism. Declarations of one's worth, nodding in agreement, these women hold space for and with each other. There is an unspoken yet known way in which we gather. It is important to note that space is not just defined by actual physical space. One can hold space with someone through empathy and compassion in the digital realm. Uniting shared stories and experiences, living in this heteronormative, patriarchal society where Black women are othered and ignored. Amen'ing and "Yes Sis" over the ways in which health and well-being has suffered as the wife, the mother, the caregiver. Having found comfort, bonds, and answers in spaces like these, I choose to write with and curate spaces for Black women to share and "be who they be." Being who we be allows for one to let their hair down and welcome vulnerability. Grounded in collective spirit and participatory soul, which is the Black woman ethos, lies my research and praxis. This ethos is rooted in the spirit of my ancestors. Within the historical trajectory of my ancestors who valued and cherished times of gatherings, both formal and informal to hold space for themselves and build community simultaneously. Gatherings were their collective ways of being and knowing. From gathering around the basin of purple hull peas needing to be picked or the kitchen or dining room table, opportunities to share and learn in a supportive, sacred spaces, women found answers within themselves and each other. Womanism forwards that notion.

The proclamation of a Womanist is grounded in liberation, self -determination, and humanity for all people. This theory bodes as a lens for consideration in addressing lived bodily experiences of African American women. Likewise, according to Bell (2019) Womanism ". . .conceptually addresses the many factors of oppression that Black women face" (p.32). Research studies from a Womanist framework have been done in the fields of education, theology, and mental health, but not within the body image field. Marr (2014) asserted, "Womanist epistemology and theory seeks to disrupt dominant ways of knowing" (p. 99). Layli (Phillips) Marpayan, Womanist scholar and researcher, has spent years researching and writing about Womanism. I find her working definition of Womanism useful:

> Womanism is a social change perspective rooted in Black women's and other women of color's everyday experience and everyday methods of problem solving in everyday spaces, extended to the problem of ending all forms of oppression for all people, restoring the balance between people and the environment/nature and reconciling human life with the spiritual dimension. (Phillips, 2006, p. xx)

The foundation of what critical scholars assert is the validity of the African American woman's experience that shapes meaning and provides wisdom. Hill Collins (1990) claimed that from an African American woman's viewpoint, "Individuals who lived through the experiences about which they claim to be experts are more believable and credible than those who have merely read or thought about such experience" (p. 209). Out of these experiences of receiving knowledge one obtains wisdom, which is verified through experience with themselves or spirit. Essentially, both scholars posit the beneficial nature of experiences. Webb-Moore (2017) stated that Womanism provides "the ability to summarize and verbalize her individual experiences as a self-defined cooperative perspective is essential to her survival" (p. 24). Espousing a Womanist consciousness demonstrates a particular stance that African American women can assert when they have been denied visibility and voice.

On a daily basis, African American women live their lives at the intersection of race, gender, sexual orientation, and class. The atrocities of physical and systemic violence inflicted upon minoritized groups such as LGTQIA+ and Black women are on the rise causing mental, emotional, and physical stress (Cataby et al., 2019; Thorpe et al., 2022). Navigating our existence in a world that chooses to ignore, tones police, sees and devalues, and silences our voices and experiences can be a challenge when one does not have community or respite spaces to be. Womanism recognizes the social construction of the African American woman's identity through a historical context which includes the legacy of slavery and the intersectionality of women's experiences (Beauboeuf-Lafontant, 2003, Vaz, 2006). Ignored, objectified, sexualized, demoralized, their lived body experiences are compared with others and/or defined for them. These narratives, experiences, and images are often times seen from the outsider perspective.

There are no studies that address the lived experiences of a Black woman's body using an arts-based approach. However there are few studies that address various aspects of the lived experience of a Black woman using various qualitative and quantitative approaches (Maynard, 2018, Capodulipo, 2015).

ARTS-BASED APPROACH BENEFITS

In discussing the benefits of an arts-based approach, Leavy (2020) states that the arts "open up new ways of seeing and experiencing and illuminate that which otherwise remains in darkness" (p.ix). This statement is particularly poignant in relation to seeing and seeking to understand the experiences of Black women and their bodies which are not fully "seen" in research studies. Arts-based research studies like Maynard (2018) offer a platform of exploration into the complexities of Black women's identities. Cole and Knowles (2008) stated:

> Art-informed research is part of a broader commitment to shift the dominant paradigmatic view that keeps the academy and community separated: to acknowledge the multiple dimensions that constitute and form the human condition—physical, emotional, spiritual, social, cultural—and the myriad ways of engaging in the world—oral, literal, visual, embodied. That is, to connect the work of the academy with the life and lives of communities through research that is accessible, evocative, embodied, empathetic, and provocative. (p. 60)

ROLE OF THE ARTS-BASED RESEARCHER

Levy (2016) asserts that the role of arts-based researchers is to shape knowledge building and transmission practices. She posits "in order to address different issues successfully and communicate effectively with diverse audiences, we need to be able to see in different shapes and to produce knowledge in different shapes" (p. 3). This approach is a great pathway to understanding a Black woman's body because it affords research participants an opportunity to bring forward a personal issue in a unique yet substantive way. Furthermore, using arts-based approaches can provide more expansive ways to bring attention to the shared experiences of Black women and girls and their bodies.

I am a PhotoArtist and Poet; in my research study, I chose to share experiences of Black women and their bodies from a Womanist, participatory researcher lens incorporating stories and images with my participants otherwise known as "sisters." In the digital, image-driven world, I purport that is arts-based approach could be advantageous in exploring the health and well-being of Black girls and women. Photography is one of the representations of the many arts-based practices scholars use to address their research questions in holistic and engaging ways. Arts-based researchers utilize methodological tools during any or all phases of the research process, including data generation, analysis, interpretation, and representation.

Leavy (2020) states that the arts "open up new ways of seeing and experiencing and illuminate that which otherwise remains in darkness" (p. ix). This approach is a great pathway to understanding a Black woman's body because it affords research participants an opportunity to bring forward a personal issue in a unique yet substantive way. Furthermore, using arts-based approaches can provide more expansive ways to bring attention to the shared experiences of Black women and their bodies. Aligned with Womanist thinking, narrative PhotoVoice methodology (Mitchell, 2011; Moletsane et al., 2007) was used in my research to allow me and the participants, my "sisters," to hear and see intimately how gender, race, and sexual orientation impact the way in which women experience their bodies. Rooted in the phenomenological experiences of women, Womanist scholars engage in discourse that troubles ideologies around women's ways of knowing and being. Phillips (2006) suggests that knowing about one's self and one's community happens at the kitchen table where "people share the truthss of their lives on equal footing and learn through face to face conversation (p. xxvii). According to Banks (2012) stories help "to answer the big questions about the meaning of life in general and our lives specifically" (p.395). Therefore the exchange of stories is an important element to the formation of ideas and Black women's ways of knowing. Story'ing "is the process used to organized discreet pieces of information about our experiences into stories which enhances our ability to remember them" (Banks, 2012, p. 395). In many homes, Black women and girls are privy to these stories that help shape their thoughts, opinions, and identity.

THE FOUNDATION

"Hold your stomach in;" "You are so cute with your chubby cheeks;" "You need to put on a girdle;" "You are thick;" "A lady doesn't clean her plate."

"From birth to nine years old, I was raised in the South. Raised in a conservative, Christian, matriarchal yet foundationally patriarchy home, many ideas around what girls and women should do, be and look like were ingrained to my fiber."

SANKOFA

At an early age, I learned the gravity of and the ideologies behind such phrases and the impact felt by not only me but many other women; Black women. I noticed that the women in my family wore girdles, "control top" pantyhose, which I recognized controlled or flattened the stomach; what could be called a uniform (Devoe, 2020). I chose to approach this work from an authoethnographic standpoint. Using an authoethnographic approach when speaking about the body is essential because it allows the researcher to interrogate one's self while critically reflecting on past experiences. . ." (Sleeter, 2020). Critical reflexivity is a key component in personal narratives that autoethnographic work produces and has the potential to elucidate much more than one person's subjective experience: "[o]ur lives are particular, but they are also typical and generalizable since we all participate in a limited number of cultures and institutions" (Ellis, 1999, p. 674). As the "sisters" in my research study shared their experiences, I journaled and captured my feelings and reflected on similar incidents that took place from girlhood to womanhood. The poem, "They." "We." is one of those reflections.

They. We.
This shit was deep
They connected
We connected
Bonding
Sharing their truth
Spoke their hidden
They saw each other
We saw each other
We heard each other
We reached forth our arms
Through our bellies to connect with each other
Conform
Resist

Freedom

One story that a participant shared in particular resonated with not only myself but several others; the experience of wearing "The Uniform." The words of all the participants were transcribed into poems. Dill (2015) utilized the participatory narrative analysis in the study that sought to "empower participants to produce texts to make sense of their lives and their home school and neighborhood contexts" (p. 128). Analyzing stories that become nuanced poems as data proffers a deeper understanding of the lived experience.

The Uniform
Panty. Girdle. Camy.
Birthed after my daughter's birth
Worn daily to conceal the rolls.
Nipped. Tucked. Smooth.
Can't go anywhere without one
Can't go anywhere without . . . a girdle
Can't go anywhere without . . . a camy
My uniform.
~ Sister Eight

Many of the sisters nodded in confirmation of liked experiences. Growing up there were ebbs and flows in the comfortability of being in my own body. Comparing myself to other girls continued into comparing myself with other women into my adulthood. "She is light skinned and skinny, that is why she has a boyfriend, and I don't," is what I would tell myself. These ruminating self-defeating thoughts related to my complexion and size led me to searching for the way to assimilate, acculturate to the Eurocentric standard of beauty; a common theme with the sisters.

38 years of not loving myself,
lack of identity, low self esteem
38 years of relying on others to define me
me. Being a dark-skinned woman.
~ Sister Three

Yo-Yo
"I already ate" I tell my parents
Skip breakfast
Wouldn't eat dinner
The cycle
Going on a diet
Working out
They would talk about my weight

THEY
Doctors... who were not African American (we went to doctors not African-American)
My MOM
"Maybe I do need to put you on a diet"
"If you want to lose weight you can"
I
know now
Black girls
Body composition is different
Different muscle mass
ways we hold fat
But .. people weren't informed back then.
~ Sister Nine

Louder voices
My parents
were the voice
telling me that I'm beautiful
telling me I'm their dark-skinned beautiful child
encouraging me to love the skin I'm in
Unfortunately
In "my community"
Spanish Harlem,
My Black brothers, sisters
Black people
Puerto Rican people
Their voices
were louder than my parents
"Blackie"
"Darky"
didn't fit in with what Black people defined as beauty.
"You Ugly!"
~ Sister Three

CONFORMING

From the weight loss franchise, Jenny Craig, to diet pills, I was on the perpetual cycle of losing weight to wear a certain size or obtain a certain weight in order to measure up to society's perception of someone who is considered "beautiful." I had the ability to present that I was confident in my body, but I really wasn't. This internalized truth haunted me for years.

Consequently, I was on a never-ending cycle to fit into a particular size. I started running in 2013. I wanted to try this as a new weight loss method when I heard of a group of Black women who ran together on a weekly basis and "no woman was left behind." Black Girls Run is a national organization started by two women to encourage Black women to run and highlight that Black women do run. Every week, there were at least three or four opportunities for women to meet up and run or walk. This supportive group encouraged, applauded, and cheered on the first woman to finish the run to the last one. No high five received by each runner would go unnoticed. While on this journey, I met women who struggled with their body image and just like me were seeking weight loss in each footstep that hit the pavement. Conversations on the roads and trails were most often about denying oneself from certain foods, extreme workout challenges, and the desire to be a certain size. This is not uncommon in exercise groups. People seek support and advice while on weight loss journeys. Unfortunately, the conversation is around altering one's appearance versus acceptance. My personal experiences with body dissatisfaction coupled with the hundreds of conversations with women in my personal and professional lives led me to query how others experience living in their melanated bodies.

Ossana, Helms, and Leonard (1992) argued that to develop a healthy identity, Black women must move from an externally and societally based definition within which women define their values, beliefs, and abilities for themselves. Black women can do that in spaces that are created for them and reinforce giving them space to share their experiences.

Using the term "healing," I elucidate Audre Lorde's (1976, 1984) work which locates healing at the center of Black women's interactions, not just with themselves, but also with others. Healing happens while porch sitting, while getting one's hair done, standing in a line at a grocery store or beauty supply shop, at the kitchen table, online community forums, or in research studies.

AGGRESSIONS

There are many forces that attack the health and well-being of Black women. These attacks come in many forms. Socially constructed ideologies about African American women found in images have been instrumental in leaving many women mentally and physically scarred (Devoe, 2020). Pejorative stereotypes projected onto women include "Mammy," "Jezebel," Sapphire," and Welfare Queen to name a few. From the iconic images of Saartjie Baartman (Gilman, 1985) to hip/hop rap music videos (African descent) women's bodies have been scrutinized and reduced to their body parts. A considerable amount of literature has been published on the sexualized perception of the African American women (Fredrickson & Roberts, 1997; Hill Collins,

1990; hooks, 1984; Littlefield, 2008; Stephens & Phillips, 2003; Szymanski & Stewart, 2010; Watson, Ancis, White, & Nazari, 2013). Black women's bodies are sites of sexual violence (Evans, 2018); violence against Black women's bodies is overlooked in the media (Williams, 2016).

There are physical and emotional wounds that are a part of the Black women's lived experience of their bodies. According to the Association for the Study of African American Life and History (ASALH), "Black Health and Wellness not only includes one's physical body, but also emotional and mental health. At this point in the 21st century, our understanding of Black health and wellness is broader and more nuanced than ever." With that being said, it is important to look at the experiences of the body differently.

Black women experience some of the most chronic forms of mental distress (Brown & Keith, 2003), largely because of the oppression experienced because of our marginalized and intersecting identities. Black women are finding and creating spaces whether virtual, digital, or in person seeking security and healing from outside attacks and gazes. This quest to find safe and brave spaces is found in the notoriety of a novel concept of doing hair and therapy (Mbilishaka, 2018). In the article *PsychoHairapy A ritual of healing through hair*, Barlow invites the reader into the *PsychoTherapy space* which is a clinical practice and theoretical orientation that links hair to mental health. "[This] lay health advisor model with stylists and barbers trains them to make mental health assessments and interventions." Centering healing and wellness, this space nourishes the mental and emotional health of Black girls and women.

In the digital space, podcasts and websites have gained popularity as platforms and places for convening conversations for and about Black girls' and women's health and wellness. *Therapy for Black Girls* is a website and podcast dedicated to Black women's mental wellness. On *The Balanced Black Girl* podcast, host Les Alfred engages with the audience the importance of mental, spiritual, and emotional health and living one's best life. The "kitchen table" has evolved and has provided wider opportunities for women to find spaces to share their stories and be in community. More intentional "kitchen tables" are needed in research projects.

REIMAGINING

As a participatory action researcher, my research intersects creative expression with qualitative data. My research proffers Narrative Photovoice (Devoe, 2020) as a viable, comprehensive, culturally relevant, approach envisioning qualitative researchers using this methodology within Black communities; advancing a unique approach to examining the health and well-being of Black girls and women. Understanding the value of communal ways Black women receive and give information is insightful for those who choose to enter research with this population. The value of collective spaces created in a participatory action research project is consistent with Few et al.'s (2003) point of view that "sharing these resources of knowledge within a safe informant defined space is empowering and useful in providing Black women a space to process their experience in a systematic manner" (p. 207). Reimagining approaches to Black girls' and women's health considers the benefit and significance of doing research with women, inviting them to capture their experiences with images and stories. Providing "virtual kitchen tables" for girls could include the creation of online spaces to meet and discuss their health and use their camera phones to document their stories. Action research design provides study participants the platform to be involved in the process (Devoe,2020).

The method and technique of PhotoVoice (Wang & Burris, 1994)—illuminating narratives triggered by and exemplified with photographs—complements the purposes of participatory action research. Reflections, stories, and photographs bring to life experiences and ideas, which further enlighten and expand the ideas, thoughts, and lived experiences of the participant. Narratives or stories are ways in which people make meaning of their lives, their world, and their culture. Historically, African Americans have a deeply rooted tradition of storytelling (Amoah, 1997). Descendants from Africa passed down this oral tradition transmitting religious customs, family and societal traditions, and cultural norms. Stories are important to understanding a person's lived experience.

Simmonds et al. (2015) reconceptualized PhotoVoice by combining narrative inquiry and PhotoVoice methodology. In essence, this method gives breadth to the voice of the marginalized group. "Its aim is to capture participants' lived experiences in the photographs they take and their reflections in their accompanying narrative" (Simmonds et al., p. 38). Photo narratives are a series of photo images accompanied by oral stories. Photos are seen as the primary source of information and the participant's account is the secondary source. Narratives offer breadth and depth to the images and to the PhotoVoice method.

Wang and Burris (1994), participatory action researchers, sought to change consciousness and inform policy with their research, particularly their method PhotoNovella. PhotoNovella, a precursor to the contemporary term PhotoVoice, is a process whereby participants are co-researchers and use their "critical data collection tool" (Bendell & Sylvestere, 2017, p. 357), the camera, to assess and elucidate issues within communities. Wang and Burris (1997) suggested that PhotoVoice,

> entrusts cameras to the hands of people to enable them to act as recorders and potential catalysts for change. It uses the immediacy of the visual image to

> furnish evidence and to promote and effective participatory means of sharing expertise and knowledge. (p. 379)

It has been suggested that in addition to eliciting rich data from participants, PhotoVoice can have a cognitive and somatic impact on individuals. Plunkett, Leipert, and Ray (2012) argued that PhotoVoice is an emancipatory health promotion practice useful as a research method to elicit rich data about the lived experience. It has been correlated with multiple mental and physical health promoting outcomes, such as empowerment and improved self-efficacy (Foster-Fishman, Nowell, & Deacon, 2005).

Envisaging consideration be given to addressing a Black woman's total body experiences into the self-care conversation is critical. A scholar practitioner, Richardson facilitates healing circles in and outside of the classroom. She argues that "in order to produce true social transformation and strive for a radical notion of collective freedom, we must pay attention not only to our individual and political/ideological positions, but also to our individual and collective practices of self-care and healing—practices that are themselves deeply political" (Richardson, 2018, p. 282). Richardson's study considered the historical conditions that addressed African American women's identity, self-worth, and well-being. As a result of facilitating healing circles,

Richardson's (2018) charge for future research was that

> scholars take into account various social processes at work in Black women's private and public lives. Family connections and upbringing, education, community, religious practices, the experience of sexual or violent trauma, and other factors may all intertwine to shape the ways in which women interpret and respond to media portrayals and representations of beauty and race. (p. 96)

Reimagining approaches to Black girls' and women's health considers how Black girls and women disrupt and negate problematic ideologies and stereotypical tropes that seek to destroy mental health. Utilizing social media platforms such as YouTube, Facebook, and Instagram to push back, coalesce, support, affirm, and defend, Bailey (2021) asserts that "Black women employ these same platforms in ways that subvert negative stereotypes through processes that can be their own health-affirming practice . . . both the process of creation and the material created are co-constitutive harm-reduction strategies" (p.11). This proliferation of "Women's digital resistance" (Bailey, 2021) demonstrates the push toward women owning spaces and using this digital spaces of sites of self-preservation.

In a research study conducted by Musgrave et al. (2022) highlighting Black Women and Femmes negative experience of harassment on social media and how they reclaim and transform their experiences into healing, participants noted despite the online harassment they were able to heal in online communities. Several of these participants found online communities that centered Black feminism and queer politics as their space of refuge. One of the participants, Niema spoke about social media's capabilities to be a part of the healing for Black women. She said "Social media can be a part of the healing by strengthening your validation and helping healing techniques that foster wellness" (Musgrave et al., 2022).

THE CALL TO ACTION

Images have been instrumental in shaping socially constructed ideologies about African American women. Images coupled with stories are powerful representations of a person's lived experience. Reflections, stories, and photographs bring to life experiences and ideas, which further enlighten and expand the ideas, thoughts, and lived experiences. When looking at an approach to consider when looking at Black girls' and women's health, I posit the use of images and stories within collective "kitchen tables" and spaces can prove to be a benefit when seeking to give voice and life to their experiences.

Hollingshead and Meggs (2022) purport that kitchen tables are "such spaces tease out an identity politics that recognizes what it means to be both Black and woman in a society that dishonors both" (p. 151). Seemingly having sacred spaces where Black girls and women are considered to be co-researchers, collaborators in sharing their lived stories disbars the notion as the research or principal investigator as the expert.

Black feminist principles delineate that women should not be objects of other people's actions as is usual in conventional scholarly research agendas. Instead, women are to be authors and authorities of their own experiences. Black women and girls as co-researchers sharing their experiences in photos and words is the future.

This call to action challenges the ways in which health professionals, researchers, and scholars do research with Black women and girls,

1. Conduct research studies *with* Black Women and girls utilizing Narrative PhotoVoice
2. Consider the "virtual kitchen tables" as research spaces where Black women and girls share their stories of healing and resilience. Finding ways to tap into a person's creativity is one of the ways to share sensitive information. Black girls from two small schools in Brooklyn, New York, who participated in Dill, Rivera, and Sutton's (2018) research, learned how to write poems to heal from relationship violence. Therefore, poetry and photography could be considered mediums or

instruments of change that can bring attention to the experiences of Black girls and women and their health.
3. Envision research studies utilizing PhotoVoice method to inform policy around Black women's and girls' health.

Understanding the value of communal ways Black people receive and give information is insightful for those who choose to enter into research with Black women. The values of collective spaces are consistent with Few et al.'s (2003) point of view that "sharing these resources of knowledge within a safe informant-defined space is empowering and useful in providing Black women a space to process their experience in a systematic manner" (p. 207).

Researchers, scholars, and public health practitioners who seek to do research concerning the health and well-being of Black women and girls must consider ancestral and contemporary ways of knowing and being that can begin at the "kitchen table."

REFERENCES

Amoah, J. (1997). Narrative: The road to black feminist theory. *Berkeley Women's Law Journal*, *12*, 84–102.

Bailey, M. (2022). *Misogynoir transformed: Black women's digital resistance*. New York University Press.

Banks, J. A. (2012). Storytelling to access social context and Advance Health Equity Research. *Preventive Medicine*, *55*(5), 394–397. https://doi.org/10.1016/j.ypmed.2011.10.015

Barlow, J. N. (2022). *PsychoHairapy A ritual of healing through hair*. https://psychcentral.com/health/psychohairapy-a-ritual-of-healing-through-hair

Bendell, K., & Sylvestre, J. (2017). How different approaches to taking pictures influences participation in a photovoice project. *Action Research*, *15*(4), 357–372. https://doi.org/10.1177/1476750316653812

Capodilupo, C. M. (2015). One size does not fit all: Using variables other than the thin ideal to understand black women's body image. *Cultural Diversity and Ethnic Minority Psychology*, *21*(2), 268–278. https://doi.org/10.1037/a0037649

Catabay, C. J., Stockman, J. K., Campbell, J. C., & Tsuyuki, K. (2019, December 1). Perceived stress and mental health: The mediating roles of social support and resilience among black women exposed to sexual violence. *Journal of Affective Disorders*, 259, 143–149. https://doi.org/10.1016/j.jad.2019.08.037. Epub 2019 August 19. PMID: 31445340; PMCID: PMC6791774.

Cole A. L., & Knowles J. G. (2008). Arts-informed research. In J. G. Knowles & A. L. Cole (Eds.), *Handbook of the arts in qualitative research* (pp. 55–70). Sage Publications.

Devoe, Y. A. (2020). In pictures and words: A womanist answer to addressing the lived experience of african american women and their bodies—A gumbo of liberation and healing. https://aura.antioch.edu/etds/611

Du Bois, W. E. B. (2008). *The souls of Black folk* (B. H. Edwards, Ed.). Oxford University Press.

Ellis, C. (1999). Heartfelt autoethnography. *Qualitative Health Research, 9*, 669–683. https://doi.org/10.1177/104973299129122153

Evans, S. Y., Bell, K., & Burton, N. K. (2018). *Black women's mental health: Balancing strength and vulnerability*. Albany: State University of New York Press.

Few, A. L., Stephens, D. P., & Rouse-Arnett, M. (2003). Sister-to-sister talk: Transcending boundaries and challenges in qualitative research with Black women. *Family Relations, 52*(3), 205–215. https://doi.org/10.1111/j.1741-3729.2003.00205.x

Finley, S. (2008). Arts-based research. In J. G. Knowles & A. L. Cole (Eds.), *Handbook of the arts in qualitative research* (pp. 71–81). Thousand Oaks, CA: Sage.

Foster-Fishman, P., Nowell, B., & Deacon, Z. (2005). Using methods that matter: The impact of reflection, dialogue, and voice. *American Journal of Community Psychology, 36*(3/4), 275–291.

Fredrickson, B. L., & Roberts, T. (1997). Objectification theory: Toward understanding women's lived experiences and mental health risks. *Psychology of Women Quarterly, 21*(2), 173–206.

Gilman, S. L. (1985). *Difference and pathology: Stereotypes of sexuality, race, and madness*. Ithaca: Cornell University Press.

Hill Collins, P. (1990). *Black feminist thought*. New Delhi: Atlantic Books.

Hollingshead, A. E., & Meggs, M. (2023). Da'Rona and a virtual kitchen table politics of community. *Black Women and Da'Rona: Community, Consciousness, and Ethics of Care*, 160.

Justin, T. A., & Jette, S. (2022). "That chart ain't for us": How Black women understand "obesity," health, and physical activity. *Health, 26*(5), 605–621. https://doi.org/10.1177/13634593211046844

Leavy, P. (2016). *Essentials of transdisciplinary research: Using problem-centered methodologies*. Routledge, Taylor & Francis Group.

Leavy, P. (2020). *Method meets art: Arts-based research practice*. The Guilford Press.

Littlefield, M. B. (2008). The media as a system of racialization: Exploring images of African American women and the new racism. *American Behavioral Scientist, 51*(5), 675–685.

Lorde, A. (1984). *Sister outsider*. Freedom, CA: Crossing.

Maparyan, L. (2012). *The womanist idea*. New York: Routledge.

Marr, V. L. (2014). Ditchin' the master's gardening tools for our own: Growing a womanist methodology from the grassroots. *Feminist Teacher, 24*(1/2), 99–109.

Maynard, K. (2018). To be Black to be a woman. Can dramatherapy help black women to discover their true self despite racial and gender oppression? *Dramatherapy, 39*(1), 31–48. https://doi-org.antioch.idm.oclc.org/10.1080/02630672.2018.1432668

Mbilishaka, A. (2018). PsychoHairapy: Using hair as an entry point into black women's spiritual and mental health. *Meridians, 16*(2), 382–392.

Mitchell, C. (2011). What's participation got to do with it? Visual methodologies in 'girl-method' to address gender-based violence in the time of AIDS. *Global Studies of Childhood, 1*(1), 51–59.

Moletsane, R., de Lange, N., Mitchell, C., Stuart, J., Buthelezi, T., & Taylor, M. (2007). Photo-voice as a tool for analysis and activism in response to HIV and AIDS in a rural KwaZulu-Natal school. *Journal of Child & Adolescent Mental Health, 19*(1), 19–28.

Musgrave, T., Cummings, A., & Shoenebeck, S. (2022, April 29). *Experiences of harm, healing, and joy among Black women and femmes on social media.* ACM Digital Library. Retrieved July 17, 2022, from https://doi.org/10.1145/3491102.3517608

Ossana, S. M., Helms, J. E., & Leonard, M. M. (1992). Do "womanist" identity attitudes influence college women's self-esteem and perceptions of environmental bias? *Journal of Counseling & Development, 70*(3), 402–408.

Phillips, L. (2006). Introduction—Womanism: On its own. In L. Phillips (Ed.), *The womanist reader* (pp. xix–lv). New York: Routledge.

Plunkett, R., Leipert, B. D., & Ray, S. L. (2012). Unspoken phenomena: Using the photovoice method to enrich phenomenological inquiry. *Nursing Inquiry, 20*(2), 156–164.

Richardson, J. L. (2018). Healing circles as Black feminist pedagogical interventions. In O. Perlow, D. Wheeler, S. Bethea, & B. Scott (Eds.), *Black women's liberatory pedagogies* (pp. 281–294). London: Palgrave Macmillan. https://doi.org/10.1007/978-3-319-65789-9_16

Sleeter, C. E. (2020). Critical family history: An introduction. *Genealogy, 4*, 64. https://doi.org/10.3390/genealogy4020064

Stephens, D. P., & Phillips, L. D. (2003). Freaks, gold diggers, divas, and dykes: The sociohistorical development of adolescent African American women's sexual scripts. *Sexuality & Culture, 7*(1), 3–49. https://doi.org/10.1007/BF03159848

Szymanski, D. M., & Stewart, D. N. (2010). Racism and sexism as correlates of African American women's psychological distress. *Sex Roles, 63*(3/4), 226–238.

Thorpe, S., Malone, N., Hargons, C. N. (2022). Black sexual minority women's social well-being and psychological distress. *American Journal of Orthopsychiatry, 92*(4), 505–515. https://doi.org/10.1037/ort0000617. Epub 2022 May 5. PMID: 35511548; PMCID: PMC9977194.

Walker, A. (1985). *In search of our mothers' gardens: Womanist prose.* New York: Harcourt.

Wang, C., & Burris, M. A. (1994). Empowerment through photo novella: Portraits of participation. *Health Education & Behaviour, 21*(2), 171–186.

Watson, L. B., Ancis, J. R., White, D. N., & Nazari, N. (2013). Racial identity buffers African American women from body image problems and disordered eating. *Psychology of Women Quarterly, 37*(3), 337–350. https://doi.org/10.1177/0361684312474799

Williams, D. R., Mohammed, S. A., & Shields, A. E. (2016). Understanding and effectively addressing breast cancer in African American women: Unpacking the social context. *Cancer, 122*(14), 2138–2149.

Chapter 7

Lifting as I Climb, Resting When I Need To

Shawn Arango Ricks

"Why is it so cold in here?" I thought to myself. I was a new department chair at the opening leadership meeting—in August—and I was freezing! I had two blankets with me, on my lap in the meeting. I was not feeling well, clearly—and yet I felt compelled to push and "make it through" this meeting. Ironically, I was knee deep in writing and researching Black women's mental health and wellness, and yet I couldn't see my own destructive behavior. I still didn't know how to rest. While I don't regret that moment, I share it honestly and openly and write about it as much as I can. As I write this more tears come up as I cry for the part of me I couldn't or wouldn't acknowledge. Couldn't see. Couldn't cherish. Couldn't love enough to allow her to rest.

I have been writing about this work for a "grip" (that's a long time in slang); however, I've been *living* this work even longer. In addition to my academic/intellectual foray into this work, I have been working as a therapist and coach with Black women, in part, around the need to let go of the Strong Black Woman (SBW) narrative (Wallace, 2009). I even wrote an article for *YES!* magazine on *How I stopped playing the Strong Black Woman.*

Black women have been subjected to three well-known stereotypes that have impacted their psychological and physiological well-being: mammy, jezebel, and strong Black woman (cite). These stereotypes, combined with gendered racism, can have a devastating impact on the overall wellness of Black women. Living up to the stereotype of the strong Black woman has become increasingly problematic. The idea of the strong Black woman arose from the groundbreaking book by Michelle Wallace, *Black Macho and the Myth of the Superwoman.* According to Wallace (1990), Black women

All the while, from a disembodied state I had not learned to acknowledge, feel, and believe that I, too, was worthy of all the things I shared through my research and writing, and with clients.

The motto of the National Association for Colored Women (NACW), *Lifting as We Climb*, has been a guiding principle for me throughout my personal and professional journey. NACW was formed in response to a clear recognition that women's groups were not meeting the needs of Blacks, and male organizations were not including women. Black women were doubly marginalized, and this unique positionality demanded a unique organization that would focus on the needs of Black women. The motto personifies the struggle of Black women's commitment to lift each other up while working on creating conditions that promote and encourage conditions that create systemic change. This principle resonated with me deeply, as I am clear that I would not have made it as far as I have without the support, guidance, and communal love of my many mentors. The elders who took me under their wing, sharing inspiration and mentoring me through environments that I didn't even always recognize as dangerous. Having a roadmap made all the difference, and I have always felt obligated to offer the same type of guidance to others. Inherently, I don't think that's where the problem resided. I think my thoughts of putting everyone before me superseded my ability to tap into some type of balance in my personal and professional life, ultimately leading me to write this.

"SHUT UP AND GIVE ME YOUR BONE MARROW"

The quote that starts this section is from a 2007 documentary by Byron Hurt I used to show in class *Hip hop: Beyond beats and rhymes*. The quote is from a time when Nelly was supposed to do a bone marrow drive at Spelman College. At the same time there was some controversy over a popular drink that one of the companies he owned produced called "pimp juice." The women of Spelman planned to protest his appearance because of his video "Tip Drill," which they believed was demeaning to women. The response to the concerns was basically, "shut up and give me your bone marrow."

It's been years since I've used this documentary in class, but this particular segment resonated with me because it reminded me of the silencing and conditional acceptance of Black women. The messages that remind us to show up—but not fully. Use our voice—but not too loudly. Be available—but don't be clingy. It's amazing to me that a lot of these messages which often show up in interpersonal relationships have woven their way into the systems in which we work and play. For me, this system is higher education.

Who Black women can be has been informed and narrowly created to allow for four main stereotypes: the mammy, the jezebel, the angry Black woman, and the strong Black woman (SBW) ((Beauboeuf-LaFontant, 2009; Ricks, 2016; Wallace, 2009; Watson & Hunter, 2015; Woods-Giscombé, 2010).

Some messaging is handed down directly: "who do you think you are?", "girl, you better get down here and help—", "only two places open after midnight: legs and the emergency room." Similarly, the indirect messaging—at least for me—was around reinforcements and rewards from when I was a "good girl." That usually equated to when I was doing well in school, being thoughtful, or helping or thinking about someone else. Conversely, I was trying hard to avoid being caught in the cross hairs of shame, blame, and guilt. I cannot remember how many conversations I overheard that shamed another Black woman for not being a martyr. Oftentimes they were subtle—the shame of the auntie who didn't like to spend all day in the kitchen. They rolled eyes at the auntie who didn't leap right up from the table and start clearing the table, grabbing plates, and starting the dish water (there was no dishwasher!). Oddly enough, this never occurred with the menfolk. In fact, it seemed as if the sole job of the women was to make sure the men were okay—was there an unspoken fear and need to keep them happy lest they leave?

This unspoken attitude, which later became an unspoken rule, was that the needs of others were far more important than the needs of self. And to focus on self—in any capacity—was selfish. As I have worked with Black women, I've noticed that there is a tendency to put others' needs before us—at all costs, meaning we will overlook warning signs and instead normalize our experiences until it is the only reality we know. I have written about this phenomenon as "normalized chaos," a defense mechanism born from the pressure of the stereotypes mentioned above that don't allow Black women to acknowledge events as I continue on my personal healing journey and work with women who are on theirs—I've realized that this perspective has come from years of societal and familial conditioning of what it means to be a "good" girl, how being "good" equals love and validation, and how busyness is a way to validate our existence.

My feeling of having to be the one to do "all the things" while simultaneously performing acts of myself (Butler, 2006) carried me from my childhood to the academy. Harley (2008) wrote about Black women being the "maids of academe" almost 15 years ago, and here I am—still echoing it. According to Harley (2008), Black women in higher education act in roles that echo many of the stereotypes mentioned above, and in doing so they end up working harder, doing the less desirable work others don't want to do, and cleaning up messes. This quote, this image of Black professional women still sweeping up after others has not left my consciousness.

MY BREAKDOWN AND BREAKTHROUGH

As I lay in bed that morning, a different type of tiredness was settling in. I did not wake up and think about the beauty of the day or notice the cacophony of the birds singing. Instead, I woke up in what I now realize was a panic. I was not sweating or hyperventilating—so to me I chalked it up to part of the chaos of my life I had normalized. I was feeling a weariness in my bones that rest was not addressing. My nervous system was in a state of hyperarousal, and I went through the motions of checking the emails on my phone and immediately felt overwhelmed. I remember not breathing. Wanting to cry but instead holding it in. I was expected in the office, at the time I was serving in an inaugural chief diversity officer position at a small, predominantly white liberal arts college. When I accepted the position, I realized that the work would be challenging; however, I underestimated the toxicity of the environment. In my 30 years of doing social justice work, the resistance to change remained high. In my role, I was geographically and emotionally isolated. The institution did not really desire change, they just wanted the illusion of change. This created an environment in which I encountered many microaggressions. The toll of the emotional labor of my tokenized role on campus was impacting my emotional, physical, and psychological well-being. Once again, I felt like a maid of the academy, doing all the dirty work no one else wanted to deal with and cleaning up faculty and staff faux pas. One of my sources of energy, student interaction, was non-existent due to the complicated nature of my appointment and the perception by students of color that I was part of the "administration." The isolation and chronic stress were taking a toll on my body and I did not have any choice but to listen. This was not like me. I used to be an early riser, and now I was barely able to get going by 9 am. That day I laid in bed all day—I didn't notify anyone I wouldn't be in—I just didn't go to the office that day. Tired, but unable to rest (what we call "wired and tired"), I wondered how I was going to keep going when my body was saying it was done. I thought about the tinnitus I had started having and the pills I needed to take just to go to sleep. I wondered how I was going to keep my relationships going when I couldn't focus on anything. It was such an unusual feeling for me because I had been able to always push through things otherwise.

The ability to "push through" was a coping mechanism I had adopted from dealing with many obstacles and adversities throughout my life. For many of the challenges I encountered, there was no option for me but to find a way to get through it–push through. Like most coping mechanisms, I overidentified with one that had been working for me unable to recognize when it was no longer a "good" choice. This phenomenon has led to some of the health disparities Black women are encountering. The historical minimization of Black women's needs and feelings has trickled into our own perceptions of who we are and what we need. As a result many Black women will keep "pushing through"--ignoring their bodies and negating their minds–until they can no longer continue. The current framing around health disparities in terms of personal ownership and compliance can partly be attributed to this mindset. Most research around health disparities oversimplifies the etymology, boiling better health outcomes to personal wellness choices–eat less pork and take more walks. This type of approach ignores the cumulative impact of chronic stress on the body, and instead adds to a culture which creates resistance and shame around prioritizing a holistic path to wellness.

I was falling into a familiar trap that Black women have silently subscribed to for generations. The irony is that, although I was able to intellectually write about wellness, I was unable to recognize conditions that were contributing to creating a state of unwellness. I had always been able to make my body do what my mind wanted, but my body was rebelling.

Of course, in hindsight, I can see the build-up happening. The meeting I referred to at the beginning of this document—the blankets in a meeting were definitely a sign. There was also the time I cried leaving the Dean's office. The irritation that I increasingly felt had finally bubbled over and although I knew this wasn't "the time or place" I couldn't stop it.

I kept saying that I was busy and *maybe* doing too much. Emphasis on *maybe*. Meanwhile there had been so many signs over the years that my daily stress was turning into chronic stress and my chronic stress was becoming burnout. Some of the things I ignored: I backed my van into the garage door because I forgot to open it; I left broccoli in the oven for 4 days; I put eggs on to boil and then left for work. Those are some of the more obvious things I ignored. Some of the more subtle things were: not having the energy to engage in physical activities that I once enjoyed, being irritable with friends, and 2 am Instagram shopping—leading me to wonder who had ordered all these wonderful packages. I had normalized the chaos (Ricks, 2018) in my personal life and disguised it as ambition and "getting it done." Once again, this was a topic I had written about—normalized chaos (Ricks, 2018)—as a coping mechanism for Black women. Revisiting that article—*my words*—I am reminded that "normalizing chaos, on the other hand, provides Black women a false sense of others' realities; thereby creating a breeding ground for toxic behaviors. When Black women start viewing their hectic, overscheduled and potentially traumatic lives as 'normal,' they continue to engage in self-defeating and unhealthy behaviors, and are less likely to recognize potential mental and physical health distress" (Ricks, 2018, p. 344). So ironic looking back that I would continue to engage in the very behaviors I was admonishing others for. At the time, I didn't fully understand the nature of trauma.

Ironically, because I became so adept at overcoming the odds and receiving kudos for doing so, it became my "go to" response. Show me something that couldn't be done and I was going to do it. Tracing back my exhaustion to being a single mother as an undergraduate at a large predominantly white institution (PWI) and taking in what I know now to be microaggressions and carrying that to pursuing (and completing) my PhD as a working mother of three—to commuting to Virginia for work. WTF.

Many times Black women are praised for being "so strong" or being resilient. At a subconscious level, this coping mechanism becomes overly relied upon and confusing. At one level, it is meeting a need to be seen and praised—even a little bit. On the other hand, showing up in one way doesn't allow for the flexibility to adjust when things are not working. It is like the old saying, if all you have is a hammer, then every problem looks like a nail.

Oddly enough, I didn't recognize any of my symptoms as burnout. I just thought I needed "a break." You know, when is spring break? When is fall break? When is winter break? In the lies I was telling myself, one of them was when "this thing happens" I would be able to rest. It seemed like those things never came, and I found myself using rest breaks to catch up on work or filling the time with some other busyness. All of which I now know are responses to trauma.

My chronic stress manifested itself in extra weight, depression, and exhaustion. I felt done with higher education, and that's when I knew I *had* to do something. As a therapist, I had encouraged Black women to take time to heal, and I have been the one to sign the paperwork. I was really familiar with the Family and Medical Leave Act (FMLA); however, I felt twinges of shame in my belly when I thought that I should take FMLA. It took me six months, and support from my doctor and therapist, to finally file the paperwork. What ran through my head prior to filing were some of the same thoughts I worked with clients on: will I be letting down my job, what will people think, is this going to impact my career? Finally, I allowed myself to take FMLA and deal with my exhaustion. Honestly, I was so triggered and used to being in a state of hypervigilance that I didn't just go home and get still. That would have been a shock to my system—like bringing a car to a dead stop on the highway. I did rest some, and scheduled lots of therapy and I also used that time to immerse myself in a healing environment. I signed up for a retreat, with some women I knew and many I didn't, a sacred sojourn to Sedona. A trip I couldn't really financially afford to take, and emotionally couldn't afford *not* to take.

That sacred retreat was the turning point for me and I returned back to North Carolina with a deeper resolve of what "self-care" and "self-love" looked and felt like. And my commitment to practice them. Mind you, prior to this trip I had been writing and researching around self-care and the importance of wellness for Black women and I had *completely* ignored myself and my needs. Completely. In the service of getting the message out, I was unintentionally inflicting harm on myself. But intention does not matter, the impact was the damaging and had long-term repercussions.

That was an important lesson I needed to learn. If I am not in the service of "self-love" what am I actually doing to myself? From a reductionist perspective, there is no neutral when it comes to how I am treating myself. Things and experiences are either in the service of my self-love and self-care or they are in the service of neglect and abuse. I heard that message when I heard bell hooks speak at a National Women's Studies Association (NWSA) conference, but you know how some messages you hear and then you don't *really* hear them for years later. Yeah. That was me.

From an epistemological perspective, I had accepted my existence as the "truth" and I was subconsciously justifying my behaviors. Everything from why I didn't have time for yoga that (or any) day to why I deserved french fries and ice cream. I had logically rationalized it in my mind that work comes first, and everything else comes second. I confirmed this position through a process of deduction by watching so many Black women before me place everything and everyone else before them. Part of the rationalization for disregarding our needs and our bodies was our passion for students and wanting to make sure students were not negatively impacted or overlooked because of some policy, among others. Our passion for helping others convinced our logical minds that it was okay to *not* help ourselves. This individual choice has been replicated so often that health issues for Black women in higher education have become more the norm than the exception.

IS IT STRESS OR BURNOUT?

This is a conversation Black women need to be having more often and more openly— recognizing the difference can be key to increasing our health outcomes, and taking our experiences—our traumas (with a big "T" and a little "t") out of the shadows removes the shame, stigma, and the perceived isolation. Believe me when I say that is why I have been brutally honest in writing and reflecting on my experiences—so much so that I have had to stop several times and regroup. We heal individually, yes—but we also heal in community. In a lot of ways writing is my virtual community.

While stress and burnout overlap in many ways, the key difference seems to be linked to duration. Stress is an adaptive response while burnout is a state of mental or emotional tiredness, which occurs out of continuous exposure to stress (Pines & Keinan, 2005). Fatigue turns to chronic exhaustion, and depression and irritability are common. Sometimes it is hard, particularly for Black women, to differentiate the line between "getting it done" and burnout. Black women have been hyping each other up to "push through" and "make it happen" and continue to wear their exhaustion as a badge of honor. Where this deeply rooted notion of not deserving to rest originated is unclear. I have often thought that perhaps it's a deeply held epigenetic knowing going back to slavery that is paradoxically rooted in self-preservation. There was no option for rest during slavery, and, in fact, to appear to be "slacking off" or being non-productive could result in physical punishment and/or emotional consequences (being sold to another plantation). As a result, what may have started as an adaptive coping mechanism continues to be handed down verbally, and in Black women's bodies. Without awareness and examination of its usefulness, this coping mechanism continues to be utilized and the thing that used to preserve us, now, in fact, is damaging—once again we are in a cycle of normalized chaos.

A gentle perspective shift could occur if Black women would intentionally, compassionately, and gently remind each other of the importance of rest. This would start with setting individual intentions to be mindful of how, or if, we are resting throughout the day. Simultaneously, engaging (or even creating) a group of women who will hold each other accountable for shared goals of rest. At a micro level, Black women can become more mindful of their individual interactions with their friends, their self-talk, their "asks" of others, and their responses when someone says "no" or they are resting. At a macro level, this could include examining messaging around rest in both the spoken and unspoken policies and examining workload and invisible labor for Black women.

EXPANDING THE DEFINITION OF TRAUMA

As mentioned earlier, shifting the narrative will demand an awareness and (re)examination of how we are showing up in the world. As I revisit my experience, I know that my use of normalized chaos as a defense mechanism was rooted in my belief in being a strong Black woman (Wallace, 1990), my own stigma around mental health and wellness, and my denial that I was traumatized. I had bought into a narrow view of trauma that did not allow me to acknowledge microaggressions and gendered racism as traumatic. According to Levine (1997) "trauma occurs when an event creates an *unresolved* impact on an organism" (emphasis mine, p. 128). Focusing on the unresolved portion of this sentence, I am once again reminded that I must first recognize experiences as traumatic before I can resolve them. How many events had I experienced that had created unresolved impacts on and in my body? Without that type of awareness, there can be no intention to make a change. As I am becoming more embodied—learning how to be more in and aware of my body—I have been offered the opportunity to resolve some of the traumas that I have experienced, but ignored or suppressed. This demands a deep dive into radical self-care and self-love, including finally learning how to rest.

Self-care and self-love that involve a deep dive must challenge the current barrage of what some might call toxic self-care that is encouraging us to shop, get massages, and treat ourselves to dinner as a declaration of self-love and self-care. While these are part of the process, radical self-care goes deeper than our purchasing power. For me, radical self-care pushes me to look at the messages I have received about deservedness (message: I must work hard to have nice things), self-worth (message: I must do things for others in order to be valued), and self-love (message: I am not worthy). Radical self-care can get ugly. It's writing—honestly—this piece, as a way to stop *performing* and start *authentically* showing up. It's allowing myself time to sit in my feelings—and feel them—without shame or judgment.

Writing has always been healing for me, starting in 7th grade when I wrote my first book of poems as an assignment. When I re-read that book, I can see how my soul was trying to peek through the dark clouds of fear and uncertainty and create a space where I could be heard. Seen. Valued. This healing journey is complex. There is often a resistance to releasing what is weighing us down. I have learned to realize that this shows up for me in resistance to writing—a passion that I have actually turned into a career (professor). I resist, procrastinate, drop projects, and so on, all as part of my individual resistance to actually having to sit with, untangle, and make sense of the background noise. The fear becomes "without the noise, who am I?" I am learning that resistance and embracing it—not as a flaw—but as a predictable and natural order of the healing process.

"WE WILL REST"

Why is it so hard for Black women to rest? Just go sit down somewhere. Put your feet up. Binge watch a show and feel zero guilt. The societal messaging discussed earlier plays heavily into this resistance; however, there are quite a number of Black women who have been writing about, advocating for, and embodying the importance of self-care and self-love for Black women as tools of liberation. Notable authors are Audre Lorde, bell hooks, Angela Davis, and Alice Walker. Many of these women remind me of the notion of "radical" self-care—meaning it is non-negotiable and it is a way to push back against white capitalism, patriarchy, and "grind" culture. We must frame this narrative of rest as a way to pay homage to our ancestors and as a liberatory tool.

The Nap Ministry, which I follow on Instagram, has been instrumental in helping me change my thought patterns and my relationship with rest.

The founder, Tricia Hersey, created the "Rest is Resistance" framework in 2016 as part of her personal healing and liberation journey. Hersey talks about healing her "generational exhaustion and racial trauma" through the use of rest. Napping then becomes a way to push back against capitalism, honor our ancestors, and get more in touch with our bodies. According to Hersey, "Black people are dying from sleep deprivation and our resistance to rest is a social justice and public health issue. Capitalism was created on plantations during chattel slavery and is the same system that is driving the entire globe to exhaustion and a deep disconnection with our bodies and minds today. We are no longer divine human beings in this system and instead machines" (2022). While the politics of Black liberation has been written about for decades, the accessibility of Hersey's Nap Ministry, with the motto of "we will rest" has motivated thousands of Black women to rethink their relationship with rest, and hopefully their relationship with themselves.

As I move more earnestly, yet compassionately, into my personal healing and wellness I am finding that reframing messages I have learned around rest and deservedness is helpful—but so is my understanding of what freedom looks like for me. I used to automatically say yes to opportunities—now I practice the pause. By practicing the pause, I mean I ask for some time to think about the request so I can decide if this "opportunity" aligns with my best and highest good or if it is in service of someone else's needs or goals. When I ask myself questions around why I overschedule, overwork, and/or overextend myself—the answers are coming from a deeper knowing. With that knowledge, I can use mindfulness to help me pause and be in each moment, be in my body, be present and . . . well, just be. My commitment to myself, my rest, and my healing is rooted in my worthiness, my deservedness, and my desire to set myself free. I enact liberatory practices from my living room couch!!

I recognize how my relationship with rest, trauma, and embodiment impacts my ability to engage in research. No matter the type of research you choose to engage in, your interpretation will be viewed through your lens. Without a commitment to interrogating messages you have received and/or believed related to worth, rest, and productivity, your research could be skewed by this unexamined view. The disconnection that comes from not knowing ourselves, honoring ourselves, and allowing ourselves to be in our body means we are not fully showing up *for* and *in* our research. For me this was all the years I have written about self-care and rest without *doing* it. I was dabbling (safely) in theory and not allowing myself to see and feel the connections and patterns both at an individual and a systemic level. Occam's razor tells us that maybe the simplest explanation or path is the one we should prefer. I couldn't agree more. Are you tired? Rest.

PHILOSOPHY OF SCIENCE

If you've gotten this far in this chapter, I suspect you are adept at cognitively knowing things and yearning to turn that knowledge into practice—this is the philosophy of science. What has worked for me, and what I share with women I work with, is the importance of understanding some fundamentals of the path we are all on. Understanding the history of how Black women learned to resist rest (and whom that benefits) and instead continue to work beyond their own wellness.

As I reflect on my journey, I am confident that I would not be this far along had I not been introduced to Patricia Hill Collins work on Black feminist thought as a foundational piece to help me understand that there were different ways of knowing and being than what I had been exposed to. Black Feminist Thought was birthed from Black movements, such as Black Nationalism, and critical social theories, such as Feminist Theory, Critical Race Feminism, Critical Race Theory (CRT), and Standpoint Theory. Black Feminist Thought is shaped by the convergence of its six distinguishing features: the dialectical relationship between Black women's oppression and activism; U.S. Black women's standpoint; connections between Black feminist practice thought and Black feminist practice; dialogical practices and Black women intellectuals; Black feminism as dynamic and changing; and the relationship between Black Feminist thought and other social justice projects (Hill Collins, 2009).

While it is important to know the "why" behind journeys it is equally important to learn how to use the intellectual portion to move us forward due to the safety of understanding versus intellectualization to paralyze us. When is enough knowledge to spur one into action? In research, we call this saturation. You have found all the information you can find on this topic. In the healing process, it is a little more complex. It's a *knowing*—a willingness and belief to take a leap and trust that you will land safely and securely.

While I leave you with some practical tips, it is my sincere hope that you will not just read them, but practice them. Start to find small ways to integrate this knowledge into your daily practice. It just takes small micro-acts of resistance to start moving you forward. Some suggestions are:

1. Do a quick mental health evaluation. If possible, see a counselor for a mental health check-up. Coping skills that may have worked for a while may need to be re-visited. It's time to reassess the difference between being *selfish* and practicing *self-care*.
2. Seek out and utilize a mental health buddy. This can be as simple as checking in with someone daily just to see how they are doing. This type of "wellness accountability check" will only work if both parties allow themselves to be vulnerable and share how they are *really* doing.

Your mental health buddy should be the person you can be honest with—and they should be honest with you.

3. Listen to your body. Our bodies are amazing at self-regulation. Things we often ignore (such as headaches and body aches) could be signals of internalized stress. Headaches, fatigue, muscle aches, and tummy troubles are just a few of the physiological symptoms of stress. Unmitigated and unreleased stress roams around the body and sends us signals for help. The tendency to overlook these symptoms and push through, because "we have to" can lead to a host of long-term chronic health problems.
4. Find time to be still. Spending 5–20 minutes a day in quiet reflection, meditation, or journaling can help reset your body's defenses. The fear of quiet and the distraction of busyness lead us around instead of the other way around. We are in charge of our minds, our time, and our overall well-being.

I wish you the best of luck on your journey. I am confident you can do it. When you feel like you need a reminder of *why* you are on this path, remember the words of Audre Lorde (1988) from her book of essays *Burst of Light:*

> I had to examine, in my dreams as well as in my immune-function tests, the devastating effects of overextension. Overextending myself is not stretching myself. I had to accept how difficult it is to monitor the difference. Necessary for me as cutting down on sugar. Crucial. Physically. Psychically. Caring for myself is not self-indulgence, it is self-preservation, and that is an act of political warfare. (Audre Lorde 1988)

REFERENCES

Beauboeuf-Lafontant, T. (2007). You have to show strength: An exploration of gender, race, and depression. *Gender & Society*, *21*, 28–51.

Butler, J. (2006). *Gender trouble*. Routledge.

Centers for Disease Control and Prevention. (2016). Health of Black or African American non Hispanic population. https://www.cdc.gov/nchs/fastats/black-health.htm.

Harley, D. A. (2008). Maids of academe: African American women faculty at predominately white institutions. *Journal of African American Studies*, *12*(1), 19–36. http://www.jstor.org/stable/41819156

Hersey, T. (2022, February 21). *Rest is anything that connects your mind and body.* The Nap Ministry. https://thenapministry.wordpress.com/

Hill Collins, P. (1990). *Black feminist thought: Knowledge, consciousness, and the politics of empowerment.* New York: Routledge.

hooks, b. (1993). *Sisters of the yam: Black women and self-recovery.* Boston: South End.

Hurt, B. (Director 2006). *Hip hop: Beyond beats and rhymes.* Byron Hurt and Sabrina Schmidt Gordon.

Junior, N. "Don't we hurt like you?: Examining the lack of portrayals of African American women and mental health" last modified May 26, 2015. https://www.bitchmedia.org/article/dont-we-hurt-like-you-black-women-mental-health-depression-representations

Lorde, A. (1982). *Zami: A new spelling of my name.* Freedom: Crossing Press.

Lorde, A. (1988). *A burst of light: Essays.* Ithaca: Firebrand Books.

Lorde, A. (2007). *Sister outsider.* Berkeley: Crossing Press.

Pines, A. M., & Keinan, G. (2005). Stress and burnout: The significant difference. *Personality and Individual Differences, 39*(3), 625–635. https://doi.org/10.1016/j.paid.2005.02.009

Ricks, S. (2015). *Psychological tight spaces: One black feminist scholar's journey into academia.* Winston-Salem: Library Partners Press.

Ricks, S. (2018). Normalized chaos: Black feminism, womanism and the (re)definition of trauma and healing. *Meridians, 16*(2), 343–350.

Valencia Jones, L., & Guy-Sheftall, B. (2015). Conquering the Black girl blues. *Social Work, 60*(4), 343–350.

Wallace, M. (1990). *Black macho and the myth of the superwoman.* London: Verso.

Walker, A. (1983). *In search of our mothers' gardens.* Orlando: Harcourt Bruce Jonavich.

Warren-Findlow, J. (2006). Weathering: Stress and heart disease in African American women living in Chicago. *Qualitative Health Research, 16*(2), 221–237.

Watson, N. N., & Hunter, C. D. (2015). Anxiety and depression among African American women: The costs of strength and negative attitudes toward psychological help-seeking. *Cultural Diversity and Ethnic Minority Psychology, 21*(4), 604.

Woods-Giscombé, C. L. (2010). Superwoman schema: African American women's views on stress, strength, and health. *Qualitative Health Research, 20*(5), 668–683.

Chapter 8

"If You Can't Relate to Me, How Can You Treat Me?"

Centering Black Girls' Voices in Culturally Responsive Health Praxis

Maryam M. Jernigan-Noesi

Overwhelmingly, Black girls have not been afforded the attention and consideration of reflecting upon, defining their health concerns, identifying facilitators and barriers to health promotion, or opportunities to contribute to recommendations that inform proposed health interventions. As reflected in the title of this chapter, and offered by a Black adolescent girl in a qualitative study designed to explore Black girls' definitions of their health and wellness (Jernigan, 2019), "If you can't relate to me, how can you treat me?" The participant highlighted the flawed and potentially ineffective thinking of health providers that assume an "objective" (i.e., universal) or color-blind ideology (denial of racial differences through an emphasis on sameness) (Neville, et al., 2013) to help facilitate ideal health outcomes for Black girls. Further, findings from the study indicated that for Black girls, a prerequisite to engaging with health providers lies in the ability of those providers to understand their developmental, socio-ecological, gender-race experiences, and other social and community factors (Jernigan, 2020). Doing so allows for health praxis that centers the experiences of Black girls and informs how they think about and approach their health. Such practice also helps to illuminate how social determinants of health—the conditions in the environments where individuals live and engage—influence health outcomes for Black girls.

PHILOSOPHY OF SCIENCE

My philosophy of science serves to reduce the application of flawed conceptions of knowledge, challenge the process of who is deemed the expert or holder of information, and dismantle the false notion of objectivity that has informed health science. As a Black woman, my social location, complex intersectional experiences, and values allow for an alternate perspective which facilitates the identification of new areas of inquiry, research questions, methods, and interpretation of findings targeting Black girls. I am a Black, cis-gendered, heterosexual, able-bodied, woman, who was raised with Christian values. As a professional psychologist, former professor, and clinical researcher, my socio-economic status has shifted throughout my lifetime. I was born into a family of six with fewer financial resources at birth than when I graduated from high school. As a graduate student, I once again navigated life with little access to adequate financial resources. My class status continues to evolve as I enter mid-career status.

When engaging Black girls, although there is a recognition that our gender-race experiences are heterogeneous, there is also a noted perception of my ability as a Black woman to accurately understand, validate, and convey the thoughts, beliefs, and behaviors of Black girls to others. This perception has afforded me the ability to inquire about and access information directly from Black girls. For example, rather than portray findings that yield health disparities between Black girls and their counterparts as a) evidence of their deficiency (Morris, 2007); b) a lack of motivation (Young et al., 2001); or c) their indifference to the importance of health (Burk, 2013), I work to elicit and center the narratives of Black girls at every level of the scientific process. This underscores the need to include Black girls as epistemic authorities and advances a liberatory and egalitarian model for health praxis.

The ideology of *womanism* (Walker, 1984) has resonated with me since I first learned of its origins while an undergraduate psychology student matriculating at a Historically Black College (HBCU). Although introduced to the concept of *feminism* as an adolescent, the depictions and narratives did not reflect my experiences or those of the girls and women of color I engaged. Feminist epistemology can be credited for illuminating the ways that gender, as a social construct, serves to inform a) our conceptions of knowledge, b) what is known and by whom, and c) practices that were used to inquire and justify knowledge (Anderson, 1995). Womanism, however, recognizes that the intricacies of identity development are informed by one's context. Unlike traditional feminist identity models (Downing & Roush, 1985) womanism represents an internal and dynamic process of racial and gender identity development for women of color, who experience differences in social power and face multiple forms of systemic oppression (Carter & Reynolds, 1996; Helms, 1990).

A FRAMEWORK FOR UNDERSTANDING BLACK GIRLS' HEALTH

For Black girls and women, womanism allows for an exploration of how predominant ideas and practices of knowledge acquisition disadvantage girls and women of color, as well as other subordinated groups or aspects of identity (Ossana et al., 1992). Moreover, womanism acts to reframe and reform such conceptions and practices to highlight the needs and interests of Black girls and women. Black girls and women have been largely excluded from health science inquiry and intervention (Beech & Jernigan, 2014). The inability for Black girls and women to serve as primary informants of their health and share their perspectives, narratives, and contributions has ultimately compromised their ability to be acknowledged as epistemic authorities of their lives. Traditional approaches to healthcare have a long history of ignoring the experiences of Black girls and women in various ways. This includes a general lack of representation of Black girls and women in clinical trials and research studies, leading to a lack of data and knowledge on how medical treatments affect them specifically. In addition, Black women's pain is often dismissed or not taken seriously by healthcare providers, leading to misdiagnosis and inadequate treatment. Such examples are detrimental to the health and well-being of Black girls and women because healthcare providers who internalize gendered and racialized stereotypes, such as the "superwoman myth," assume that Black girls and women are strong (i.e., can handle more pain). This leads to healthcare decisions that negatively impact their treatment (e.g., less pain management and less empathy). In essence, health providers may hold implicit biases that affect their decision-making and treatment recommendations, leading to unequal treatment and outcomes for Black women. The aforementioned represent a legacy of historical trauma that Black girls and women have, and continue to face relative to their healthcare. Other examples include a history of medical experimentation and the long-standing mistreatment of Black individuals in the United States, which has created a legacy of mistrust of the medical system. Such factors are critical in reframing the narrative and underlying assumptions that are often presented as a lack of healthcare utilization and compliance with recommended treatment plans for medical services. In other words, Black girls and women are not underutilizing healthcare services or ignoring the recommendations of health professionals. The healthcare system often fails to consider and meet their unique needs and experiences.

As such, Black girls and women are subjected to healthcare practices and policies that lack essential knowledge about their unique experiences. Healthcare providers therefore are likely to lack the knowledge, skills, awareness to meaningful engage Black girls and women. They are less likely to investigate appropriate content and explore health-related information through questioning that considers important factors in their lives correlated with their health and well-being.

Consequently, predominant theories and conceptualizations that have informed health science are not inclusive or representative. As such Black girls and women are invisible, thus reinforcing social hierarchies and oppression.

My focus on centering Black girls' narratives to inform health science and praxis is rooted in a desire to disrupt the use of the concept of *universality* as the standard and ideal metric by which others are compared. Universality—the notion of similarities that exist among individuals—is more often based on the experiences of the status quo group in a given society. In the context of the United States, Black girls' health and health outcomes are often descriptively compared racially to White youth and Black boys (Epstein, Blake & Gonzalez, 2017). As such, Black girls are neglected in the writings of researchers and scholars because they tend to treat Black girls as analogs of Black boys. When gender is considered in research studies, Black girls are most often compared to white girls (LePage, 2021). There is an overwhelming obliviousness to their experiences and a scarcity of health science that focuses specifically on the challenges of being a Black girl. Despite continued documentation of racial and gender health disparities when Black girls are compared to their racial and gender counterparts (e.g., overweight, obesity) they have rarely been the sole focus of health science research or praxis. Therefore, interventions designed to foster health and well-being remain scarce (Beech & Jernigan, 2014).

Situated knowledge. The information, knowledge, and experiences of Black girls reflect their unique gender-race identity perspectives. Additionally, other aspects of identity that intersect with Black girls' gender-race identity help to situate what is *known* and how it is *known* (i.e., what influences the perspective of Black girls). Black girls are the *knowers* of their firsthand experiences and sense of self, given the context in which they exist and attempt to thrive. They are the primary source for reflecting upon how they experience the world and how they perceive the world experiences (i.e., embodiment). When engaged and afforded the opportunity, Black girls express their emotions, attitudes, and beliefs based on their unique perspectives. The ability of others to be informed of, and by, Black girls' knowledge lies in the proximity and quality of the relationship. The absence of such relational connections has been noted and insight may lead to the aforementioned erroneous and misguided interpretations (e.g., Black girls do not care about their health).

As a consequence of how society has devalued the lives of Black girls, minimal attention has been given to the specific challenges they face and how such barriers are associated with their coping (Thomas, Hacker, & Hoxha, 2011; Evans-Winters, 2007). Coping, from a behavioral health perspective, is an essential factor in helping to further explore how the unique challenges Black girls face, may facilitate or serve to deter their health and well-being (Jernigan, 2019). To develop interventions aimed at enhancing Black girls' ability to identify and utilize their existing strengths as an informer of health prevention and intervention, it is first necessary to examine Black girls' gendered and racialized experiences within a social and cultural context (Brown & Jones, 2004; Cokely, 2006; Spencer, 2005; Tyson et al., 2005).

Embodiment. Understanding Black girls requires one to recognize and validate their social location. Black girls are mistreated in a manner consistent with racial and gender stereotypes, each of which is equally salient and negatively evaluated by society (Ward, 2006). Further, Black girls' gender-race-class socialization outside of their immediate caretaking environment occurs informally and in relation to the systems they engage (e.g., school, community). Historical and current accounts have highlighted that the environments in which Black girls exist rarely promote positive identity development or self-concept (Morris, 2007; Rollock, 2007; Shorter-Gooden & Washington, 1996). To buffer such experiences, Thomas and King (2000) argue that appropriate socialization messages for Black girls should include historical information about racial oppression and its influence on gender roles. The concept of gendered-racial socialization embodies the messages that are implicitly and explicitly communicated to Black girls related to dual experiences of racism and sexism that Black girls and women face (Thomas & King, 2000). Knowledge about what is missing from the gender-racial socialization experiences of Black girls, offer opportunities to counter messages that they may receive about themselves. Given the presence and impact of external factors, such as social media, on Black girls' perceptions of themselves and their social location, health providers who are unaware or minimize such information, risk loss of an opportunity to increase awareness and engage (i.e., relate) to Black girls.

Social and Cultural Context. As indicated previously, the experiences of Black girls are often contrasted to Black boys (Epstein et al., 2017). Comparing Black boys and girls makes invisible the unique challenges and realities faced by Black girls and is ultimately misleading (Saunders, Davis, Williams, & Williams, 2004; Ward 2006). As Ward (2006) posits "It is not that Black girls are doing so much better, but that Black boys are simply doing much worse" (p. 225). More recent scholarship underscores this point, highlighting the fact that many Black girls continue to encounter barriers to their health and well-being (Epstein et al., 2017; Morris, 2015).

Schools, as microcosms of society, appear to be particularly inhospitable settings for Black girls. They spend approximately 30 hours per week in school (Sturm, 2005), which makes academic settings a significant influencer of their development (Morris, 2007; Rotheram-Borus, Dopkins, Sabate, & Lightfoot, 1996; Van Galen, 1993). As reflected in society, educational environments likely incorporate meanings of race and gender that undoubtedly parallel race-gender attributions at a societal level (Cokley, 2006; Morris, 2007; Saddler, 2005; Tennant, 2006). As such, scholars note that Black girls are often treated in a manner consistent with societal racial and gender stereotypes (Crenshaw, 2015; Ward, 2006; Shorter-Gooden & Washington, 1996). Jernigan (2009) reported that Black girls in school settings frequently encountered racism and sexism. Such biases were often reflected by several negative outcomes including increased referrals by school administrators for behavioral concerns and precipitous declines in the girls' academic performance. Additionally, Morris (2007) found that educators often treated Black girls more negatively than any of their other race or gender counterparts. Findings suggest that although Black girls' demonstrated interest in learning and engagement in school, teachers explicitly encouraged other students, but negatively evaluated Black girls and labeled them as aggressive when they were outspoken.

Despite the aforementioned challenges, Black girls are often applauded for their resilience, especially relative to educational outcomes (U.S. Census Bureau, 2004). Because of the seeming academic success of Black girls in education (e.g., graduation rates), emphasis on their resilience is often highlighted as a source of personal strength (Evans-Winters, 2007; Shaffer, Coffino, Boelcke-Stennes & Masten, 2007). This characterization is problematic in that reviews of the risk and resilience literature pertaining to youth of color more often describe resilience as adaptation despite the risk (Arrington & Wilson, 2000). Nicolas et al. (2008) and Jernigan and Daniel (2011) reject the notion of resilience as it pertains to Black youths. The notion of resilience, as it pertains to Black girls, highlights the positive outcomes of some yet assumes that their normative cultural context is predominantly negative (Nicholas et al., 2008). Such deficit-based and pathologizing models often used to describe the condition of Black girls do not employ a strengths-based approach, which highlights the positive factors inherent in Black culture that leads to the healthy development of Black girls.

Alternately, Nicolas et al. (2008) proposed that providers consider the coping strategies that Black girls may utilize to deal with barriers to their development and optimal functioning: withdrawal, resilience, and resistance (see table 8.1). *Withdrawal*, the first strategy, is described as the removal of the individual from stressful stimuli. Withdrawal is exhibited psychologically by detaching mentally and/or emotionally from situations that are perceived as threatening, and through disengagement with institutions (Morris, 2007; Paul, 2003). Whereas *resilience* is a passive response motivated by external

Table 8.1 Black Girls' Coping Strategies

Strategy	*Definition*	*Characteristics*	*Examples*
Withdrawal	Removal of the individual from stressful stimuli	• Black girls psychologically detaching mentally or emotionally from situations that are perceived as threatening • Disengagement from institutions	• Black girls minimizing health concerns and not following up with health providers • Perceived lack of compliance with health recommendations
Resilience	Passive response to stress or oppression motivated by external factors	• Black girls described as "bouncing back" from adversity. • Ability to "absorb" and cope with change, oppression, or difference	• Black girls who maintaining academic grades and adhering to institutional standards despite health concerns due to experiences of marginalization and social determinants of health
Resistance	Internally motivated strategies used to resist oppression	• Requires critical awareness and the ability to analyze situations to facilitate action	• Black girls requesting more diverse health providers to facilitate health education and provision of services • Black girls questioning and challenging health providers about their use of formal medical terminology to explain health concerns

factors, *resistance* is internally motivated and requires critical awareness, the ability to analyze situations to facilitate action, when necessary (Nicolas et al., 2008; Robinson & Ward, 1991; Watts et al., 2003; Ward, 2007). This conceptual thinking allows for a more accurate strengths-based model (Nicolas et al., 2008). Black girls who attain "success" as measured by societal constructs (e.g., educational attainment) are not *resilient*, but rather embody the ability to *resist* barriers that they encounter in the various environments in which they exist. Development of resistance is necessary for Black girls in particular, because they are engaged in the process of identity formation in settings that are replete with racial and gender marginalization (Robinson & Ward, 1991). Such processes require awareness and intentional effort. Therefore, Black girls' responses should be interpreted as active vs. passive and as reflective of their need to be prepared to engage a society that requires a critical consciousness, skills, and strategies to combat subjugation.

Conceptualizing Black girls' health requires the ability to identify their potential areas of vulnerability in order to connect them with resources and support systems. Taking into consideration the social and cultural context of Black girls allows for the identification of risk factors (e.g., discrimination), which are associated with poor health outcomes (e.g., increased weight, emotional distress) (Shaffer et al., 2007). On the societal level, Black girls are being referred to juvenile courts and detained in juvenile settings at disproportionately high levels when compared to girls from other racial or ethnic backgrounds, which creates a consistent pattern of overrepresentation. More specifically, Black girls face incarceration rates six times higher than those of their peers (Stefurak & Calhoun, 2004). They are becoming the fastest-growing segment of the juvenile justice system with more severe sentences when they are detained (Crenshaw, 2015). In the late 1980s and 1990s, Black girls experienced an 80% increase in juvenile detention (Eller, 2002). This trend has continued over time (National Academy of Sciences, 2000; Stefurak & Calhoun, 2004).

The experiences of Black girls are rarely documented and represent a relatively new dimension in health science and praxis. Despite some study in this area, when the literature on Black girls is considered collectively, it appears that there is very little information about how Black girls can resist barriers and challenges that they may encounter. To address the limitations of existing health science and praxis that target Black girls, there is a need to explore questions about the influence of experiences that they encounter on their health and development. Research on Black girls and resistance to oppression highlights the importance of understanding the ways in which Black girls actively resist oppression in their daily lives. Black girls resist gendered racism and other forms of oppression in their lives in a variety of ways. For example, what is encompassed in the notion of "Black girl magic" includes recognition of Black girls' resistance through their creative expression including the arts, music, or writing that showcases their experiences and perspectives. Black girls also resist oppression through their efforts to build and sustain community. Black girls (and women) are often noted as being the pillars of their communities. Such practices may involve curating safe spaces or groups for support in their neighborhoods and communities, developing virtual communities to foster connection, and their engagement with community-based projects or agencies. Black girls resist oppression in their daily lives when interacting with the various systems they must engage in, such as schools. Therefore, they resist oppression by seeking out opportunities to expand their knowledge, awareness, and education. This includes participating in educational experiences that empower them to understand the history and evolution of their oppression, while developing strategies for resistance. Resistance to oppression for Black girls is demonstrated through their activism and advocacy as well. They may engage in protests, organizing, and advocating for systemic change by challenging policies that attempt to reinforce inequities. Finally, Black girl resistance is reflected in Black girls' practice of self- and collective care. Black girls resist oppression through individual and collective activities that allow them to prioritize their overall health and well-being. This may include practices such as meditation, engaging in physical activity to reduce the impact of stressors, or seeking mental health support.

The aforementioned perspective and examples differ from the more commonly discussed concept of resilience, which focuses on the ability to bounce back from adversity. Black girls' resistance involves their ability to challenge and subvert oppressive structures and systems, as well as their ability to find joy and pleasure in the midst of adversity. It is essential to center the unique experiences and perspectives of Black girls, and has highlighted the need for health interventions and policies that support their resistance and empowerment. By shifting the focus from resilience to resistance, one is able to access a more nuanced and comprehensive understanding of the ways in which Black girls navigate and resist oppression in their lives.

REIMAGINING HEALTH PRAXIS FOR BLACK GIRLS

To address the health needs of Black girls, health providers must begin to integrate an understanding of their experiences, which offer a contextual schema to assess and make recommendations for treatment intervention. Such a framework will allow health scientists and practitioners to identify multi-dimensional areas for intervention (e.g., institutional, systemic) rather than the tendency to treat individuals as if they are the sole source of influence of their health. In other words, centering Black girls' experiences allows clinicians to inform the immediate need for care, as well as work to dismantle structural barriers that may deter health and development.

Framework. Jernigan (2020) proposed a conceptual framework that uses a socio-ecological model approach to highlight the complex nature of individual, relational, community, societal, and cultural-historical factors that influence Black girls' health. Doing so a) allows for greater awareness of factors that may compromise or promote health outcomes; b) increases the likelihood of offering feasible and culturally responsive health-promoting behavioral strategies; c) ensures that health praxis considers relationships that serve as supports for Black girls; and d) considers the social and community-level factors that facilitate or deter health outcomes.

Health praxis should prioritize salient aspects of Black girls' identity across multiple domains and integrate such factors into health praxis. For example, at the individual level, recognition of Black girls gendered-racial history and experiences helps to integrate discussion regarding resistance strategies as a means of coping with the discrimination they encounter in society and the institutions they engage. In doing so, Black girls are ideally able to utilize health-promoting coping strategies to resist oppression in its many forms (e.g., systemic) (Helms, 1990; Thompson & Carter, 1997).

Relationally, Black girls often observe or seek the guidance of Black women to inform their thoughts and beliefs about health (Jernigan, 2019). As such, engaging Black women and other adults are essential given they rely on the adults around them for access to resources that facilitate ideal health outcomes (e.g., nutrition, financial resources). At the social and community level, Black girls' health relies on accessible and equitable healthcare. The inability to attain such access can impede the ability to reduce or eliminate documented health disparities for Black girls. Ensuring the health agencies, providers, and resources exist in the places and spaces that Black girls occupy helps to enhance their ability to engage and maintain their health. Schools, faith-based organizations, and community agencies offer ideal partnerships to increase healthcare access for Black girls. Healthcare providers collaborating with such institutions help to facilitate continuity related to health messaging in support of the health and wellness of Black girls.

Holistic Health Intervention. Black girls' health requires a holistic approach. Black girls do not represent a monolith. As human beings, their health needs and concerns are multi-faceted. Employing a multidisciplinary team of providers and integrated care models allows for multiple perspectives and areas of expertise to address health. Black girls are more likely to present for annual health exams in primary care settings. Therefore, ensuring the availability of specialty care providers to address related health concerns decreases the need for multiple visits to access such providers and facilitates coordinated care. For example, previous health models have emphasized attention to health behaviors as a primary influencer of health outcomes. As such emotional and behavioral health are often treated as ancillary factors. Understanding the relationship between emotional and behavioral health to physical health outcomes allows for an integrated approach to care. Providers and health agencies who integrate behavioral health specialists are better able to identify mental health issues that may influence or exacerbate health issues.

Recommendations. To best execute use of the proposed framework for health praxis for Black girls, healthcare provider should specifically consider the following factors.

- Address biases: Healthcare providers should engage in ongoing training that allows them to identify and address biases they may hold. As research has illustrated, such biases contribute to disparities in care for Black girls. Regular self-assessment, bias training, and a commitment to equitable treatment can help
- Use racially conscious and culturally responsive frameworks to engage. Providers must take responsibility and remain accountable for continued education on the importance of cultural factors that illuminate the specific needs of Black girls in order to better understand and address their health concerns.
- Employ active listening and empathy. Engaging in active listening and demonstrating empathy can help establish trust and rapport with Black girls. This involves paying attention to their concerns, validating their feelings, and acknowledging the impact of their gendered, racialized, and intersectional experiences on their overall well-being.
- Focus on providing patient-centered care. Patient-centered care considers the individual needs, preferences, and values of Black girls. This includes involving them in decision-making processes and ensuring they feel heard and respected throughout their healthcare journey.
- Emphasize communication. Culturally responsive communication techniques take into account the linguistic, social, and other cultural contexts of Black girls. This includes using language that is respectful, inclusive, and free from stereotypes. Because individuals are not often aware of the implicit attitudes and beliefs they may hold until they are recognized by another person who provides them with feedback, continuing education initiatives that provide ongoing training opportunities and skill development are ideal. This allows healthcare providers to move beyond the cognitive and intellectual notion of cultural consideration to developing concrete strategies and skills when engaging with Black girls.
- Engage in collaborative care. Collaborate with other healthcare providers, community organizations, and support systems to create a network of care that Black girls can more easily access.

CONCLUSION

Black girls have rarely been the focus of health science and praxis despite well-documented health disparities (Beech & Jernigan, 2014). Addressing the needs of Black girls requires that health scientists and practitioners reframe the approach to engaging and treating Black girls' health. Centering the narratives and experiences of Black girls allows for a holistic approach to promoting their ideal health and development. Thus, reimagining Black girls' health requires increased awareness regarding their individual, relational, community, societal, cultural, and historical experiences. This foundational knowledge becomes the basis for determining the ways in which socio-ecological factors influence Black girls' health, health behaviors, and health outcomes. In doing so, health praxis is better able to appropriately assess, address, and advocate for Black girls' health and wellness through prevention and intervention methods that incorporate their unique experiences.

REFERENCES

Anderson, E. (1995). Feminist epistemology: An interpretation and a defense. *Hypatia, 10*(3), 50–84. https://doi.org/10.1111/j.1527-2001.1995.tb00737.x

Beech, B. M., & Jernigan, M. M. (2014). Is that all there is? A comprehensive review of obesity prevention and treatment interventions for African American girls. In V. M. Brenna, S. K. Kumanyika, & R. E. Zambrana (Eds.), *Obesity interventions in underserved communities: Evidence and directions* (pp. 63–76). Baltimore, MD: Johns Hopkins University Press.

Burk, B. N. (2015) Black girls' perceptions of health and ideal body types. *Journal of Gender Studies, 24*(5), 496–511, https://doi.org/10.1080/09589236.2013.856750

Carter, R. T., & Parks, E. E. (1996). Womanist identity and mental health. *Journal of Counseling and Development, 74*(5), 484–489. https://doi.org/10.1002/j.1556-6676.1996.tb01897.x

Cokley, K. (2006). The impact of racialized schools and racist (mis)education on African American students' academic identity. In M. Constantine & D. W. Sue (Eds.), *Addressing racism: Facilitating cultural competence in mental health and educational settings* (pp. 127–144). Hoboken, NJ: John Wiley & Sons Inc.

Crenshaw, K. (2015). *Black girls matter: Pushed out, overpoliced and underprotected.* Center for Intersectionality and Social Policy Studies. Retrieved from https://www.atlanticphilanthropies.org/wp-content/uploads/2015/09/BlackGirls-Matter_Report.pdf

Downing, N. E., & Roush, K. L. (1985). From passive acceptance to active commitment: A model of feminist identity development for women. *The Counseling Psychologist, 13*(4), 695–709. https://doi.org/10.1177/0011000085134013

Epstein, R., Blake, J., & Gonzalez, T. (2017). Girl interrupted: The erasure of Black girls' childhood. *Center on Poverty and Inequality Georgetown Law.* Retrieved from https://www.law.georgetown.edu/poverty-inequality-center/wp-content/uploads/sites/14/2017/08/girlhood-interrupted.pdf

Jernigan, M. M. (2007, December). *Managing race and culture in schools*. Presented at the Annual Metco Director's Association Conference, Norwood, MA.

Jernigan, M. M. (2019). "Why doesn't anyone help us?": Therapeutic implications of black girls' perceptions of health. *Women & Therapy*, *42*, 343–324. https://doi.org/10.1080/02703149.201

Jernigan, M. M. (2020). Exploring Black girls' recommendations for healthy lifestyle interventions to address obesity. *Journal of Pediatric Psychology, 45*(8), 887–899. https://doi.org/0.1093/jpepsy/jsaa062

LePage, B. (2021). *In schools, Black girls confront both racial and gender bias*. FutureEd McCourt School of Public Policy Georgetown University. Retrieved from https://www.future-ed.org/in-schools-black-girls-confront-both-racial-and-gender-bias/

Morris, E. W. (2007). "Ladies" or "Loudies"?: Perceptions and experience of Black girls in classrooms. *Youth and Society, 38,* 490–515.

Neville, H., Awad, G., Brooks, J., Flores, M., & Bluemel, J. (2013). Color-blind racial ideology theory, training, and measurement implications in psychology. *The American Psychologist*, 68, 455–66. https://doi.org/10.1037/a0033282

Ossana, S. M., Helms, J. E., & Leonard, M. M. (1992). Do "Womanist" identity attitudes influence college women's self-esteem and perception of environmental bias? *Journal of Counseling and Development, 70,* 402–408.

Rollock, N. (2007). Race, gender and achievement Why Black girls don't matter: Exploring how race and gender shape academic success in an inner city school. *Support for Learning, 4*, 197–199.

Rushton, P. J., & Jensen, A. R. (2005). Thirty years of research on race differences in cognitive ability. *Psychology, Public Policy, and Law, 11*(2), 235–294.

Shorter-Gooden, K. (2004). Multiple resistance strategies: How African American women cope with racism and sexism. *Journal of Black Psychology, 30,* 406–425.

United States Census Bureau. (2004). Table 7 Educational attainment of the population 25 years and over by sex, for Black alone and White alone, not Hispanic: March 2004. Retrieved February 9, 2008, from www.census.gov/population/www/socdemo/race/black.html.

Walker, A. (1984). *In search of our mothers' gardens: Womanist prose*. San Diego: Harcourt Brace Jovanovich.

Ward, J. V. (2006). Uncovering truths, recovering lives: Lessons of resistance in the socialization of Black girls. In B. Leadbeater & N. Way (Eds.), *In urban girls: Resisting stereotypes* (2nd ed). New York: New York University Press.

Young, D. R., Gittelsohn, J., Charleston, J., Felix-Aaron, K., & Appel, L. J. (2001). Motivations for exercise and weight loss among African-American women: Focus group results and their contribution towards program development. *Ethnicity & Health, Aug-Nov 6*(3–4), 227–245. https://doi.org/10.1080/13557850120078143. PMID: 11696933.

Chapter 9

Using the Guided Hair Autobiography for Black Women and Girls as a Health Assessment

Afiya Mbilishaka

"I don't get it." I was on my second interview for a tenure-track faculty position at a historically Black college in an unairconditioned cement-colored classroom in the psychology department. Small circles of sweat began to condensate on my Black blazer on top of my African print blouse that my mother purchased in Nigeria during her first trip to the continent in the early 1970s. I breathed in slowly and deeply to erase the frustration in my voice after carefully crafting my research talk to the small group of clinical psychology faculty about my emerging practice of "PsychoHairapy." My mind was retracing each recruitment step that led to this very interview. I had already written about how PsychoHairapy was utilizing hair as an entry point into mental health services for Black women in my meticulously written cover letter. I had already explained PsychoHairapy was training barbers and hairstylists in mental health first aid during the initial phone interview the previous week. At this point in the evaluation of my program of research in the interview, I was screaming in my head "What don't you get?!" as I re-stated my research interests. The interview committee was composed of one White woman in her 70s, three Black women in their 40s and 50s, and one Chinese immigrant male in his 50s. My eyes begged the other Black women in the room to explain what I was talking about to the Chinese immigrant male as he made the comment after my research presentation, "I don't get it." He repeated, "I don't get how hair is related to mental health. I simply do not understand how there can be a connection between these variables."

I did not get . . . the job.

Western Psychology has indoctrinated faculty and students to oppress Blackness through research and clinical practice (Auguste et al., 2023). According to Auguste and colleagues (2023), Black people have historically been left out of psychology research due to systemic racism and the perpetuation of harmful stereotypes. Researchers have often relied on biased samples and failed to account for the unique experiences and perspectives of Black individuals. This has resulted in a limited understanding of mental health in the Black community and a lack of culturally sensitive treatments. Additionally, the unethical history of medical experimentation on Black people in the United States has created a deep mistrust of the medical establishment, making it difficult to recruit Black participants for research studies (Washington, 2008).

It's important to acknowledge that the exclusion of Black women from psychology research has had significant consequences. The lack of representation has led to a limited understanding of mental health in the Black community and has resulted in a lack of culturally sensitive assessments and treatments for Black women. I have felt compelled to address this issue. As a researcher, I am attempting to improve the representation of Black women in psychology research using community-based participatory research (CBPR). This approach involves partnering with Black community members to design and conduct research studies that are relevant and meaningful to their experiences (Smith et al., 2015). Anecdotally, we know that hair matters in the lives of Black women. By involving Black women in the research process, CBPR can help to build trust and establish a sense of ownership over the research on hair and mental health. I see my mission to actively recruit Black women as participants and ensure that studies are accessible and culturally sensitive. I developed recruitment strategies that are tailored to the Black community (Mbilishaka, Coffen & Lacey, 2018), such as partnering with community organizations and utilizing social media platforms to reach potential participants.

In my faculty interview, I did not have any research evidence that supported my claim that there was a relationship between hair and mental health for Black girls and women. It became my mission over the next six years to develop a rigorous and inclusive method to explicitly connect concepts that I knew to be true in my life and the lives of my Black girl and women clients. I needed methodological tools. I needed evidence that could speak louder than me. I needed the voices of Black women to explain the connection between hair and mental health.

Black women have long been marginalized in academic health research, often being excluded from studies, or treated as a homogenous group. Africana womanism, a theoretical framework developed by Hudson-Weems (1993), offers a unique perspective that centers the experiences of Black women. It acknowledges the impact of colonialism, racism, and sexism on Black women's lives and recognizes their agency in resisting these forces. African womanism also values community, spirituality, and the interconnectedness of all things, which aligns with many Black women's cultural values. Using African womanism as a theoretical framework allows Black women to conduct research that is representative, empowering, and reflective of their experiences, especially as it relates to hair (Mbilishaka, 2018a).

African womanism (Hudson-Weems, 1993) is now my framework for academic research. I believe that it allows Black women to address the historical marginalization they have faced in academia. By centering the experiences of Black women, this theoretical framework acknowledges the unique challenges we face due to the intersectionality of their identity. African womanism (Hudson-Weems, 1993) recognizes that Black women have agency in resisting the forces of colonialism, racism, and sexism that have historically oppressed them. Furthermore, the values that Africana womanism prioritizes, such as community and spirituality, align with many cultural values held by Black women. This allows for a more holistic and culturally relevant approach to research that reflects the experiences and perspectives of Black women. In addition to centering Black women's experiences, Africana womanism (Hudson-Weems, 1993) also encourages collaboration and interconnectedness. This approach emphasizes the importance of building and maintaining relationships within communities, which can lead to more meaningful research that truly reflects the needs and experiences of Black women. Overall, using Africana womanism as a theoretical framework for research not only empowers Black women but also allows for more accurate and representative studies that reflect our experiences and perspectives.

THE PATHWAY OF AN UNCONVENTIONAL CONSTRUCTIVIST

I must have missed the days in my research methods class where we covered philosophy of science. I am not sure if this is a memory block on my part or if I genuinely was not there during my undergraduate and graduate studies that focused on philosophy (I doubt that I missed the class, because I made sure to get my money's worth by never skipping class). As a research-scientist and a Black woman, I often do not rely on existing philosophies from textbooks that only feature White males, but turn inward to do what Cal Newport (2016) calls "deep work." I rely on myself. I study myself. I am curious about who I am. I have decided that if a health or mental health topic is important to me, then it could have relevance to other Black women, and if others are not intrigued by an issue, then the topic is still relevant to "a" Black woman and that still fits within the realm of science.

My approach to research is a bit unconventional. I do not focus on labeling variables at conceptualization. I have decided that I want techniques, skills, and practicality when addressing the needs of my therapy clients. I believe my research training as a clinical psychologist always relates back to how to assess, diagnose, and intervene on matters of mental health. I decided to train under Black research-scientists and was formed in the margins. Although I had a breadth of courses in psychology and sociology during my undergraduate studies, Black women were never at the center of the questions under investigation. I needed a space to explore research questions that interested me as a Black woman and to be open to making mistakes, misunderstanding the research process without having to fear that others would view it because of my race or gender, and to be able to sit comfortably in confusion and excitement.

I decided to attend a historically Black university for graduate school. Before going on my graduate school admissions interview, I had never seen an entire classroom filled with Black students AND a Black professor on a college campus. I can remember staring into the lecture hall door window and gasping at a sea of Black intellectuals. This was in contrast to my undergraduate institution, where I was often the only Black student in my entire class and I never had a Black professor in psychology. I joyously decided to attend Howard University.

As a Black woman, getting a PhD in clinical psychology can be crucial in serving the mental health needs of other Black women. This is because Black women face unique challenges and experiences that are often overlooked or misunderstood in traditional mental health settings. By having a deep understanding of the cultural and societal factors that impact the mental health of Black women, a clinical psychologist can provide more effective and culturally responsive care. Additionally, having more Black psychologists can help to reduce the stigma around seeking mental health services within the Black community. Overall, obtaining a PhD in clinical psychology can be a powerful way for Black women to empower themselves and their communities.

The curious graduate student in me began to question, "What is reality?" and "How can I examine this reality?" I came to the personal conclusion that there are multiple realities, and that knowledge can be interpreted to understand the underlying meaning. I now understand this to be a constructivist approach to research.

Using constructivism in analyzing narratives in psychology can be helpful for several reasons. Constructivism is a theory that emphasizes the role of the individual in constructing their own understanding of the world around them. This is particularly useful in analyzing narratives, as narratives are inherently subjective and shaped by the experiences and perspectives of the individual telling the story. By using a constructivist lens, psychologists can better understand how individuals construct meaning through their narratives, and how those meanings shape their understanding of themselves and the world. Additionally, constructivism allows for a more nuanced analysis of narratives, as it recognizes that multiple interpretations of a story can be valid depending on the individual's perspective. Overall, using constructivism in analyzing narratives provides a more holistic and nuanced understanding of the role of narrative in psychology.

When analyzing a narrative using constructivism, it is important to understand that knowledge is not simply acquired, but rather constructed through personal experiences and interactions with the world. To begin the analysis, consider the different perspectives and experiences of the characters in the narrative, as well as the social and cultural contexts in which the events take place. Next, examine the ways in which the narrative constructs and reinforces certain beliefs or values, and consider how these might be challenged or subverted. Finally, reflect on your own personal experiences and how they might influence your interpretation of the narrative, and be open to engaging with alternative perspectives and interpretations.

Race narratives are crucial in studying the lives of Black women as they provide insights into the unique experiences of this population. Black women face intersecting forms of oppression due to their race and gender, resulting in distinct social and political realities. By examining race narratives, researchers can better understand how Black women navigate and resist these oppressive systems, illuminating the complexity of their lives. Furthermore, centering Black women's voices and experiences in research challenges dominant narratives that have historically silenced and marginalized this group. Overall, incorporating race narratives into the study of Black women's lives is essential for a comprehensive understanding of their experiences and the development of effective strategies for social change.

DEVELOPING THE GUIDED HAIR AUTOBIOGRAPHY

My graduate school studies focused on narrative personality psychology. I was a member of a research lab that studied race narratives—stories that centralized race meaning in identity development. It was in the Identity and Success Research Lab, at Howard University, that we studied hundreds of these race narratives to help to inform the theory of Race Self Complexity (Winston et al., 2004). Race self-complexity argues that race adds an additional layer to constructing the narrative of self. This theory is an extension of the work of Dan McAdams's (1997) life storytelling model. To elicit self-defining life stories, McAdams formulated an instrument entitled, "The Guided Autobiography." This instrument consisted of eight prompts of specific episodic memories across the life span, including earliest memory, childhood memory, adolescent memory, nadir, high point, turning point, continuity, and morality.

It becomes the task of the participant to construct narratives that have a clear beginning, middle, and end, a negotiation of feelings, a setting, and coherent theme or major takeaway from the experience as relates to their personality.

My research advisor, Dr. Cynthia Winston-Proctor, and fellow graduate student lab member, Dr. Tanisha Burford, curated a race-related tool to direct participants in the construction of race narratives. The instrument was birthed in 2005 and entitled, "The Guided Race Autobiography" (GRA). Using McAdams's GA, Burford and Winston-Proctor included race in each prompt of the GRA. For example, the earliest memory prompt transitioned to the earliest memory of race prompt. This new tool was piloted for my master thesis. The central research question for my thesis asked: What is the thematic content and emotional tone of the earliest memories of race of Black college students? My thesis findings suggested that cultural racism was the most common theme and fear was the most frequently represented emotion in earliest memories of race for Black college students (see Mangum, 2006). Further, my dissertation findings extended this emotional density research to address how it feels to be Black in American society and culture (see Mangum, 2010). The majority of the race narratives from adolescent memories of race centralized intense anger that continued to linger at the time of the oral or written telling of the race experience. These findings were helpful as I trained further in narrative therapy and developed strategies that utilized the GRA for race narrative therapy (Mbilishaka, 2018b).

My interest in making a connection between hair and mental health was informed by my race narrative research. I observed several race narrative episodes written by Black female college students to focus on hair. Participants narrated experiences when they felt like they were mistreated because of their hair or that they were socialized around being a Black woman through a hair-related experience (see Wilson, Mbilishaka & Lewis, 2018).

I developed my own measurement tool for hair and identity. I adapted the Guided Autobiography and Guided Race Autobiography for hair. In 2014, I started the PsychoHairapy Research Lab at Howard University, and I was on a mission to construct my own guided autobiography on a topic that I cared deeply about as a Black woman. I created the Guided Hair Autobiography (GHA; Mbilishaka, 2014). This tool elicits narratives about lived experiences across the life span related to hair. I created prompts requesting stories about the earliest memory of hair, the low point or "nadir" for hair, and a turning point in how the individual thought about their hair. For example here is one of the prompts in the exact wording for the earliest memory prompt:

> Every story begins somewhere and stories about your hair are no exception. Your earliest memory might be considered the beginning of your hair story. This may be an experience involving a family member doing your hair, your

> first trip to a salon or barbershop, or even being teased about your hair at school. Please think as far back in your life as you can. Choose from your distant memory what you consider to be your earliest childhood memory involving hair for which you are able to identify: what happened, who was involved, what you were thinking, and what you were feeling. Give us your best guess of your age at the time of the event. In addition, please speculate as to why this event is significant in your hair story and how it shaped you as an individual.

These prompts elicit narratives about hair ranging from topics of entertainment, education, economics, labor, law, politics, sex, religion, and health.

HAIR, HEALTH AND HERITAGE STUDY

The psychology of hair refers to the study of the psychological and emotional impact of hair on individuals. It explores how hair can influence self-perception, social interactions, and even career opportunities. Our hair is often seen as an expression of our identity and can play a significant role in our self-esteem. As such, understanding the psychology of hair can be useful in a range of fields, from marketing and advertising to healthcare and counseling. For example, hairstylists can use this knowledge to help their clients feel more confident and positive about themselves, while psychologists can use it to better understand how hair-related experiences can impact their patients.

The Hair, Health, and Heritage Study was the first research study to include the GHA. This study was a mixed-method research study designed to elicit hair stories and connect these hair stories with popularized measures of racial identity and mental health inventories. The study was approved by multiple institutional review boards at universities in the Washington, DC metropolitan area. I decided that I wanted to collect data with my psychology research team in the Washington, DC metropolitan area Black hair salons and barbershops. With this digital survey, the full survey questions could be digitally shared and completed in any space. On average, participants took 40 minutes to complete it. The data was collected from racially diverse groups (although the intention was to focus on Black people, all races could complete the survey). Data collection took place between February 2017 and February 2018.

Here is a sampling of data analysis of the GHA data with a focus on barbershops:

> To analyze the data, the web-based surveys were saved onto Microsoft Word documents, deidentified, and password protected by the principal investigator. Because all of the stories were responses to a digital survey, there was no transcription needed. The "find" function within Microsoft Word was used to finalize the sample from the larger data set; all of the stories in this sample

> had to include the term barbershop, barber, or shop. The text that referenced barbershops were cut and pasted into another Microsoft Word document. Using Braun and Clarke's (2006) approach to thematic analysis, the data were analyzed to identify patterns and interpret overlapping topics in the narrative data. As with all rigorous qualitative data analysis of lived experiences, trustworthiness needed to be established (Lincoln & Guba, 1985). This multirater system established credibility through a systematic audit trail of raw data and coding. The data analysis therefore occurred in six stages for the research team. Stage 1 included an initial read to gain familiarity with the stories (see Braun & Clarke, 2006). It was during this stage that analytic notes were first taken, and digital markings were made on the documents for preliminary ideas for codes. Familiarization included three reads of each story. Stage 2 focused on composing a list of salient terms and topics through a line by line read to see if there were overlapping described experiences about the hair care process. Using a table on a Microsoft Word document, researchers performed an exploratory analysis to organize brief descriptions of what was being said in the hair stories to specific terms. Terms like community and family emerged as initial codes to describe who was featured in the hair stories, as gendered racial socialization was central to the research agenda. Stage 3 included the grouping of the topics and organizing them into themes with accompanying written code definitions and names related to how Black men processed and engaged meaning making of family and community dynamics (see Braun & Clarke, 2006). Here, terms like family and community were grouped based on the psych-emotional responses based on acceptance and rejection by family and community members. Stage 4 consisted of establishing coherence and clarity between the themes. During this stage, behaviors were distinguished from emotions, leaving "ritual" as a behavior to be separated from feelings, such as "belonging" or "distress." A code book was written and used to code the narratives. Stage 5 included refining the names of themes used in Stage 4, making sure that the name matched the essence of the theme to tell a coherent story about Black men in barbershops or with barbers. The code book was revised accordingly. Finally, Stage 6 amounted in producing a report. Each theme was finalized in a digital file with direct quotes from participants to exhibit the findings. These themes may serve as a reference for future studies about Black men and hair. This disclosure of the data analysis and the narrative sampling offers credibility via quotes from participants. (Mbilishaka et al., 2021, p. 5)

PUSHING FORWARD TO BECOME A HAIR HISTORIAN

Hair is a complex language system that can communicate age, marital status, health, wealth, and career path (Byrd & Tharps, 2014). I had to develop a skillset as a historian to be able to analyze hair narratives. I read every book that I could find on the culture and history of hair. Byrd and Tharps's (1999) "Hair story" was my entry point into a deeper processing of the timeline of

Black hair in America. I first read the book during my third year of graduate school. I unpacked thousands of years of history looking for follicles. Hair was used for rituals across the African Diaspora for healing (Mbilishaka, 2018a). Rituals are a strategy to prepare the mind, body, and spirit to receive a blessing (Somé, 1998). From baby naming ceremonies to burial rituals, traditional African healers using hair follicles or decorate the hair with adornments to channel spiritual energy (Byrd & Tharps, 2014). These traditions were lost in translation during the Transatlantic Slave Trade and colonization on the African continent (Morrow, 1990). Hair became weaponized for Black women in particular, as hair was deemed as "wool" or "fur" to dehumanize our ancestors. These messages of hair trauma were passed down between generations and can be seen in current hair care practices and internalized texturism (Mbilishaka, 2021).

I have focused on studying African hair rituals. These hair rituals are life giving and centralize the health of Black women and girls. It is a way that we can more deeply connect with ourselves, African history, and our African ancestry. I consume several African history books every year and I am always on the lookout to add a ritualistic fact to my medicine bag. African rituals often include health behaviors, such as praying, singing, dancing, and even cooking. Studying rituals in Africa is crucial as they play a significant role in shaping the culture and beliefs of African communities. Rituals are often used to mark important events such as births, deaths, and marriages, and they provide a sense of continuity and identity within these communities. Through the study of rituals, we can gain insights into the social and political structures of African societies, as well as their religious and spiritual beliefs. Additionally, the study of rituals can help us understand the ways in which African cultures have evolved over time and how they have been influenced by external forces. Overall, the study of rituals in Africa is essential to gaining a deeper understanding of the diversity and complexity of African societies and their cultural heritage.

Hair has been used for millennia to evoke spiritual energy of protection. The Maasai of today's Kenya and Tanzania use several methodologies to evoke protection of newborns, brides, and warriors. During the baby naming ceremony, a Maasai family will wait seven to ten days after a baby is born to address concerns like infant mortality, waiting for the safe arrival of family members from far out villages, and to complete a personality assessment of the newborn baby (Beckwith & Fisher, 1999). During this baby ceremony, the hair of the mother and the hair of the baby are shaved off carefully with a razor blade. This is a method to ensure the health of the child in the first few weeks and months of life. The hair is understood to be so sacred that the cutting of the hair is a payment to the spiritual realm. Hair is literally currency to the gods! Hair is the highest point on our entire bodies and therefore the most connect with the divine (see Byrd & Tharps, 2014). Additionally, Masai warriors must grow locs. This loc process serves to strengthen connection with environment for space perception and comradery. Also, they must dye their hair a bright red color using paint and clays from the earth. This bright red color is used to evoke the warrior energy of the gods, such as those deities that govern blood and fire (Beckwith & Fisher, 1999). Also, when a Masai bride gets married, she must completely shave her hair. This process prepares her to enter into the marriage as a new woman, free of the stress and emotional debris of the past (Beckwith & Fisher, 1999).

Studying the healing methods of our African ancestors is important for several reasons. First, it allows us to understand and appreciate the rich cultural heritage of African societies. Second, it provides insight into the holistic approach to healthcare that was prevalent in these societies, which can inform modern medical practices. Additionally, studying these healing methods can help to bridge the gap between traditional and Western medicine, promoting cultural sensitivity and inclusivity. Finally, it can empower members of our communities to take control of their own health and well-being by drawing on the knowledge and practices of their ancestors.

Many of the healing methods used by African ancestors were based on natural remedies and plant-based medicine, which can be a more sustainable and eco-friendly approach to healthcare. Understanding the cultural context of these healing methods can also shed light on the social and spiritual aspects of health in African societies. By recognizing the value of traditional healing methods, we can also challenge the dominant narrative that Western medicine is the only legitimate form of healthcare. This can be especially empowering for marginalized communities who may have been excluded from Western medical systems. Studying these healing methods can also inspire innovation and new forms of interdisciplinary research, as scholars and practitioners seek to bridge the gap between traditional and modern medicine. For example, some researchers are exploring the potential of integrating African herbal medicine with modern pharmacology to create more effective treatments for diseases. By promoting the study and preservation of African healing methods, we can contribute to the broader project of decolonizing knowledge and promoting cultural diversity in academia and beyond. Hair care could be a key to this process.

GOING TO HAIR SCHOOL

It is important for Black women to go to hair school because it allows them to gain specialized knowledge and skills in caring for and styling Black hair. This training can lead to better job opportunities, higher income potential, and the ability to provide quality services to their clients. Additionally, by attending hair school, Black women can also become advocates for proper hair care and debunk harmful stereotypes surrounding Black hair. Overall, hair school can provide a strong foundation for a successful career in the beauty industry and empower Black women to elevate their skills and expertise.

It is important for Black women to specialize in caring for natural hair for several reasons. First, natural hair has unique properties that require specialized knowledge to maintain and style properly. Additionally, the mainstream beauty industry has historically marginalized and excluded Black women and their hair, leading to a lack of resources and expertise in caring for natural hair. By specializing in natural hair care, Black women can empower themselves and their communities while also promoting self-love and acceptance of Black hair. Furthermore, providing specialized services for natural hair can create economic opportunities and help to break down systemic barriers in the beauty industry.

I had to get trained as a hairstylist in order to be a PsychoHairapist and a culturally informed researcher that honored community-based participatory research. After earning a PhD in clinical psychology, I still wanted to learn more. I decided to enroll in hair school. I spent a year taking course work and an applied practicum. I styled the hair of over 100 Black women to complete my certification. I was under the supervision of hair care professionals and was graded on the quality of my service and styling. I rushed between lecture halls and shampoo bowls, between office hours and blow dryers. I imbedded myself into a forced ethnographic study to learn the language and skills of hair care.

DEVELOPING A HAIR AND MENTAL HEALTH CURRICULUM

Hairstylists often have close relationships with their clients, who may share personal information or concerns during their appointments (Mbilishaka, 2018b). Therefore, it is essential that hairstylists are trained in Mental Health First Aid (MHFA) to recognize signs of mental health issues, provide initial support, and refer clients to appropriate resources. Mental health issues can have a significant impact on an individual's well-being, and early intervention can lead to better outcomes for mental health care. With MHFA training, Black hairstylists can play a crucial role in promoting mental wellness and reducing the stigma surrounding mental health. This can ultimately benefit both clients and the hairstyling industry.

Hairstylists give good advice because they have developed a close relationship with their clients over time (Mbilishaka, 2018a). They often spend hours with their clients, listening to their stories and concerns while working on their hair. This creates a unique bond that allows hairstylists to understand their clients on a deeper level, including their personal style, preferences, and lifestyle (Linnan & Ferguson, 2007). Additionally, hairstylists are trained professionals who have in-depth knowledge of hair care, styling techniques, and product recommendations. They can offer expert advice on how to maintain healthy hair, the best products to use, and how to achieve a desired look. Overall, hairstylists are a trusted source of advice and guidance for their clients, making them an invaluable resource for anyone looking to improve their hair care and styling routine (Neil & Mbilishaka, 2019).

With the completion of my education as a hairstylist and after the data collection of thousands of hair stories, I decided to develop a PsychoHairapy certification. Through research-informed findings about Black women, hair, and mental health, I curated a curriculum and teach classes on how to use hair as an entry point into mental health services for Black women. This 12-hour course covers the history of our hair, the science of Black hair, mental health first aid applications, and oral and written exams.

As a clinical psychologist, I was trained to assess, diagnose, and intervene on matters of mental health. I noticed a racial disparity in my field, "most Black [people] who experience psychological distress do not receive mental health services because the dominant model of service delivery is often inaccessible and culturally disengaged" (Mbilishaka, 2018a, p. 382). My teaching, research, and service are fueled by building knowledge about the impact of oppression on the lives of people of the African Diaspora, viewing Black psychological perspectives as a source of strength, and embracing African aesthetics. I specialize in unraveling the impacts of racism through the meaning of hair. To inform this program of research and clinical practice, I completed training as a hairstylist and developed research methods to amplify hair stories and hair care spaces in the scientific literature in psychology.

To methodize this approach to the health of Black women and girls, I've intentionally trained my students to ethically engage in the collection of community data in Washington DC metropolitan salons and barbershops (Mbilishaka, Coffen & Lacey, 2017), and through social media (Neil & Mbilishaka, 2019; Davis, Mbilishaka & Templeton, 2019). Integrating a theoretical framework of narrative psychology and racial identity, we developed qualitative methodological strategies, data analytic techniques, and clinical practices. Essentially, we have innovated a global mental health and hair movement: PsychoHairapy. We developed core arguments and then disseminated our findings to the Association of Black Psychologists and American Psychological Association members through their conferences and their journals. Our findings highlighted the attachment styles and racial socialization related to hair within families (Wilson, Mbilishaka & Lewis,

2018; Mbilishaka, Mitchell & Conyers, 2020) and intimate relationships (Mbilishaka, 2018c). The most impactful application of this work with students and faculty on a national level was through the CROWN Act (Creating a Respectful and Open World for Natural Hair; and anti-discrimination bill related to hair), with our focus on the early childhood aesthetic traumas in schools and then larger society (Mbilishaka & Apugo, 2020; Mbilishaka, Clemons, Hudlin, Warner & Jones, 2020; Apugo, Mawhinney & Mbilishaka, 2020). We now have evidence that hair salons and barbershops can be sites for healing from racism and psychological distress (Mbilishaka, 2018b; Mbilishaka, Mbande, Gulley, & Mbande, 2021). This work has been internationally recognized, making several voyages to Havana, Cuba, for service learning, data collection, and dissemination (Mbilishaka, Ray, Hall & Wilson, 2020).

My two avenues of research are revealed in published writings. The articles and chapters that treat the issues related to Black hair grapple with matters of well-being, diagnosis, and intervention. When treating oppression's psychological consequences, the writings of Drs. Frantz Fanon and W.E.B. Du Bois loom large. Both were non-psychologists, but they called our attention to the impact of racism on body images and body schemas. I extend the work of these pioneers and chart the sometimes rough, sometimes smooth contours of the history and psychology of *hair* among women of African descent—the most despised of *the damned* in western society. It is risky indeed to take on this topic. Sadly, the field is much more comfortable with conversations about stereotype threat or cultural normlessness.

My research work sketches the dimensions of an unrelenting attack on the Black body. Most of my papers take advantage of the power of qualitative methods. In my hands these methods lay bare complicated consequences for intra- and interpersonal relationships that grow from the hair aesthetics the West has promoted. I had to lean into becoming a methodologist. Many, but not all my papers study the hair issues in women of African descent in the United States. Indeed, with the Guided Hair Autobiography, I show the deep-seated nature of the internalized western views of people around the globe. Even in international progressive settings the bias against Black hair persists.

The findings from the systematic study in *Media Psychology Review* of images found in *Ebony* magazine provide a historical view that is at the same time, enlightening and distressing. Again, these findings point to racism's persistence. However, my use of qualitative methods also uncovers ways that Black women create hair institutions and spaces where resistance to and transformation of racist input are born. These spaces house promise for the intergenerational healing of wounds and the promotion of growth in Black communities. In this respect, the body of work created from the Guided Hair Autobiography provided moves beyond the descriptive to the prescriptive.

Hair becomes "an entry point into psychological services" (Mbilishaka et al., 2017; Psych Discourse).

All these studies have been used to support the CROWN Act, which stands for "Creating a Respectful and Open World for Natural Hair," and it is a law that prohibits discrimination based on hair texture and protective styles such as braids, twists, and locs. The Act is designed to protect individuals who have been targeted and discriminated against due to their natural hair in the workplace and other public places. The law has been passed in several U.S. states and cities, making it illegal for employers and schools to discriminate against people based on their natural hair. The narrative elicitation of Black hair from the Guided Hair Autobiography is one of the primary sources for this bill. Little did I know that the rejection from a tenure track position could alter the laws of the United States.

CONCLUSION

Using hair for healing fits within the framework of Africana Womanism—being an outgrowth of an African cultural schema that focuses on the matchless reality, difficulties, demands, and aspirations of women of African descent (Hudson-Weems, 1993). Although Africana Womanism articulates the significance of a range of themes from an Afrocentric and anti-sexist perspective, this chapter extends the themes associated with self-definition through enlivening existing community-centered mental health interventions embedded in the authentic bonds of sisterhood and nurturing in the Black hair salon setting. The objectives of this written contribution are to reinforce Africana Womanism (Hudson-Weems, 1993) in order to: (a) illuminate the historical role of hair in healing; (b) dislocate westernized conceptualizations of mental health by articulating African spiritual rituals; and (c) embolden those whose approach addresses the intersections of healthcare and hair care. Africana Womanism frames the needs of Black women through our unique relationship to hair to address mental and spiritual health. The elicitation of narratives about hair can further guide the deeper exploration of the health and lives of Black women.

REFERENCES

Beckwith, C., & Fisher, A. (1999). *African Ceremonies*. Ann Arbor, MI: Harry Abrams.

Braun, V., & Clarke, V. (2006). Using thematic analysis in psychology. *Qualitative Research in Psychology*, 3, 77–101. http://doi.org/10.1191/1478088706qp063oa

Byrd, A., & Tharps, L. (2014). *Hair Story: Untangling the Roots of Black Hair in America*. New York: St. Martin's Press.

Davis, D., Mbilishaka, A., & Templeton, T. (2019). From "about ne" to "about we": Therapeutic intentions of Black American women's natural hair blogs. *Journal of Social Media in Society*, 8(1), 105–123.

Hudson-Weems, C. (1993). *Africana Womanism: Reclaiming Ourselves*. Troy, MI: Bedford Publishers.

Linnan, L., & Ferguson, Y. (2007). Beauty salons: A promising health promotion setting for reaching and promoting health among African American women. *Health Education & Behavior*, 34(3), 517–530. https://doi.org/10.1177/1090198106295531.

Mangum, T., Mbilishaka, A.,& Apugo, D. (2019). Protective styles: Aesthetic trauma and support inclassrooms for Black girls. *Psych Discourse*, 53(1), 8–10.

Mbilishaka, A. (2018).Black lives (and stories) matter: Race narrative therapy in black hair carespaces. *Community Psychology in Global Perspective*, 4(2), 22–33.

Mbilishaka, A. (2018).PsychoHairapy: Using hair as an entry point into Black women's spiritual andmental health. *Meridians: Feminism, Race & Transnationalism*, 16(2),382–392.

Mbilishaka, A. (2018).Strands of intimacy: Black women's narratives of hair and intimaterelationships with men. *Journal of Black Sexuality and Relationships*,5(1), 43–61.

Mbilishaka, A. (2019).Statement on behalf of the association of Black psychologists on the need forhair anti-discrimination laws. *Psych Discourse*, 53(1), 6–7.

Mbilishaka, A. (2020).Adorning Black bodies: Race narrative therapy in black hair care settings. *Journalof Contemporary Narrative Therapy, Release,* 3, 2–3.

Mbilishaka, A. (2021).PsychoHairapy: Brushing up on the history and psychology of Black hair. *Eyeon Psi Chi*, 25(3), 26–29. https://doi.org/10.24839/2164-9812.Eye25.3.26

Mbilishaka, A., &Apugo, D. (2020). Brushed aside: African American women's narratives of hairbias in school. *Race Ethnicity and Education*, 23(5), 634–653.https://doi.org/10.1080/13613324.2020.1718075

Mbilishaka, A., Clemons,K., Hudlin, M., Warner, C., & Jones, D. (2020). Don't get it twisted:Untangling the psychology of hair discrimination within Black communities. *AmericanJournal of Orthopsychiatry*, 90(5), 590–599. https://doi.org/10.1037/ort0000468

Mbilishaka, A., Coffen, P.,& Lacey, C. (2017). "Don't harm a hair on their head": Culturallymeaningful and ethical psychological data collection in black hair care spaces.*Psych Discourse*. Retrieved from http://psychdiscourse.com/?view article&id 690:feature-2&catid 294:feature-articles-v51-2

Mbilishaka, A., Mbande, A.,Gulley, C., & Mbande, T. (2021). Faded fresh tapers and line-ups: Centeringbarbershop hair stories in understanding gendered racial socialization forBlack men. *Psychology of Men & Masculinities*, 22(1), 166–176.https://doi.org/10.1037 /men0000317

Mbilishaka, A., Mitchell,D., & Conyers, C. (2020). Grandma's hands: Memories of hair stylinginteraction with African American grandmothers. *Journal of*

IntergenerationalRelationships, 18(2), 139–155. https://doi.org/10.1080/15350770.2019.1658008

Mbilishaka, A., Ray, M.,Hall, J., & Wilson, I. (2020). 'No toques mi pelo' (don't touch my hair):Decoding Afro-Cuban identity politics through hair. *African and BlackDiaspora: An International Journal,* 13(1), 114–126. https://doi.org/10.1080/17528631.2019.1639298

Mbilishaka, A. M. (2014). *TheGuided Hair Autobiography [Data collection instrument].* Washington, DC:Howard University.

Mbilishaka, A. M., &Lacey, A. (2019). Don't sweat your hair out: The frequency of exercise forAfrican American women with natural hair. *Journal of Exercise and Nutrition,*2(1), 4–11.

Mbilishaka, A. M., &Mbilishaka, T. (2018). Wakanda trick is This?: The deeper psychologicalconsequences of disney's the Black Panther. *Sankofa: Pan African Journal ofNation Building and ReAfrikanization*, 28, 86–93.

Neil, L., & Mbilishaka, A. (2019). "Hey curlfriends!": Hair care and self-care messaging on Youtube by Black women natural hair vloggers. *Journal of Black Studies*, 50(2), 156–177.

Smith, T., Mbilishaka, A., & Kennedy, K. (2017). Press and curl: An examination of ebony magazine covers to understand the cultural-Historical trends of Black women's hair. *Media Psychology Review*, 11(1).

Smith, S. A., Whitehead, M. S., Sheats, J. Q., Ansa, B. E., Coughlin, S. S., & Blumenthal, D. S. (2015). Community-based participatory research principles for the African American community. *Journal of the Georgia Public Health Association,* 5(1), 52–56.

Wilson, I., Mbilishaka, A., & Lewis, M. (2018). "White folks ain't got hair like us": African American mother-daughter hair stories and racial socialization. *Women, Gender, and Families of Color*, 6(2), 226–248.

Chapter 10

Breaking the Concrete Ceiling

Shifting and Stress Among Black Women in the Workplace

Danielle Dickens

INTRODUCTION

Due to the double marginalization of being Black and a woman, many Black women in the United States experience being the "token," or one of few, Black women in the workplace. As a result, the standard to judge and measure Black women's behaviors and thoughts becomes consistent with the white dominant culture, making it difficult to decipher between what is racist and what is normal behavior of the dominant culture (e.g., Tatum, 1987). As a token, Black women may be subjected to more experiences of discrimination and heightened levels of visibility while also being invisible due to the marginalization of being Black and a woman (Dickens, Womack, & Dimes, 2019). Due to being tokenized in the workplace, Black women may feel the need to engage in certain coping strategies, such as identity shifting as a form of survival in predominantly white spaces, such as the workplace. Identity shifting refers to the unconscious or conscious process of altering one's speech (code-switching), behavior, appearance, and perspectives (Dickens & Chavez, 2018; Jones & Shorter-Gooden, 2004). As an example, Black women may shift between speaking standard American English to "sound white" in predominantly white workspaces to fit in and/or to avoid experiencing racism, and speaking in African American Vernacular English outside of work.

Though shifting may assist Black women, across different career statuses, advance in their career, it can take a psychological toll on Black women who may feel pressured to alter important aspects of their identity in the workplace, such as their attire or natural hair style. Thus, shifting has been found to be associated with higher levels of stress, anxiety, and depressive symptoms among career-oriented Black women (e.g., Jones et al., 2021). More attention should be made to the stressors associated with Black women's engagement in code-switching and shifting of their appearances and perspectives. The goal of this chapter is to highlight literature on how early career and senior career status Black women engage in shifting as a coping strategy to experiences of workplace discrimination and discuss the health outcomes associated with shifting. This research has implications for how employers can build a culture of inclusivity which lessens the need for Black women's engagement in identity shifting.

MY POSITIONALITY

As a Black feminist social psychologist and my identity as an educated Black woman who has engaged in identity shifting influenced the way I approach research in the area of shifting. The experiences of racism and sexism in graduate school forced me to navigate through the higher education institutional system as a modified self to survive psychologically and physically in a predominantly white institution and environment. Currently, I am a tenured associate professor at a women's historically Black college. My personal experiences with discrimination and identity shifting within and outside of academia are what led me to research this topic on shifting and relevant outcomes of shifting. I also utilize interdisciplinary research and theories to explore this research. In all, I aim to contextually center the lived experiences of Black women to identify effective strategies to reduce health inequities and to improve their career development.

HAIR AND SHIFTING

Due to societal norms, women in general are pressured to focus on their body image, including their appearance (Watson, Lewis & Moody, 2019). Based on Black women's gendered racial identity, Black women attribute significant meaning to being Black and woman. Black women's hair is an important part of their identity (Jones & Day, 2018). In recent years, the criminalization of natural hair through discriminatory school and workplace policies has received considerable attention (Opie & Phillips, 2015). For example, in 2014, the U.S. Army updated their AR 670-1 policy which prohibited traditional African American hairstyles (e.g., locs, braids, twists). However, there are policies that have been recently passed to circumvent this discriminating act. As such, the *Creating a Respectful and Open World for Natural Hair (CROWN) Act of 2020* is a California law that prohibits discrimination based on a person's hair texture or hairstyle if that style or texture is commonly associated with a particular race or national origin among those participating in federally assisted programs, housing programs, public accommodations, and employment. Yet, still many states in the United States can legally discriminate against someone based on natural hair styles.

Black women's hair, which includes afros, braids, coils, locks, and natural curls, has been in the media headlines lately. As an example, a Black woman in Louisiana was fired for wearing her natural hair instead of a wig (Fowler, 2021). As such, Imani Jackson put a cap over her naturally curly hair and glued a wig with straight hair in its place, every day. One day, she stopped wearing the wig and instead began wearing her natural hair in a bun and within a month, she was fired (Fowler, 2021). There are other countless stories of Black women and girls being teased for, excluded from, and disciplined at school and/or work because of their Black natural hairstyles (Rogers, 2021). Consequently, Black women may alter their hairstyles; for instance, when preparing for an interview by wearing their hair straight instead of in a natural hair style to avoid discrimination by not getting a job offer because of their hair style. When Black women are not able to be their authentic self in the workplace, by wearing hairstyles as they wish, it can be taxing and lead to stress.

COLORISM

Another body image factor that might influence Black women's engagement in shifting and related stress is colorism. Colorism refers to the preference for lighter skin which is closest to Eurocentric standards of beauty (Lemi & Brown, 2020). Colorism is a type of racialized gendered standard of beauty that dates back to slavery and is a result of internalization. There is this notion that there are better outcomes or "light skin privilege" due to colorism, such that lighter-skinned Black people were more likely than their darker-skinned counterparts to have more years of education, higher salaries, and more prestigious jobs (Hughes & Hertel, 1990). This is one example of the ways in which colorism is systemic and illustrates how pervasive color-based preference is within our society (Harrison, 2010; Hill, 2000).

Based on previous research, it can be implied that colorism for Black people, in particular Black women, has significant consequences for the experiences of Black women in the workplace. As such, since colorism is the preference for lighter skin, which is associated more with Eurocentric standards of beauty, lighter-skinned Black women may be viewed as more likable to their white counterparts (Harrison, 2010; Hunter, 2002). Furthermore, research has found that Black people as a whole are more attractive when they have physical features, such as skin color, hair texture, nose, that most resembles Eurocentric rather than Afro features (Hill, 2002; Maddox & Gray, 2002). More specifically for Black women, a study found that lighter-skinned Black women had more job satisfaction regarding pay and career advancement compared to their darker-skinned Black women colleagues (Catalyst, 2001). Due to these beauty standards, many Black women attempt to hold themselves to them though these beauty norms are often impossible for even white women to achieve. Moreover, Black women may shift by surgically changing their features to conform to the standards of beauty. These findings highlight the key role that skin color can play for Black women in the broader society in general and in the workplace in particular.

CAREER STATUS AND SHIFTING

Another factor that can impact Black women's engagement and stress associated with shifting is their career status. Based on research by Thomas et al. (2013), women of color, in particular Black women, may experience what is known as the "pet to threat" phenomenon at various career stages. For instance, when Black women enter their career, they may be perceived as a pet by being asked to do minor tasks. However, as they advance in their careers, they will be perceived as a threat and may experience harsher forms of discrimination (Thomas et al., 2013). This *pet to threat phenomenon* may impact how Black women across different career stages experience discrimination and cope with experiences of discrimination in predominantly white workspaces. As Black women enter their career, there may be pressure to alter their appearance to advance in their career. As such, it is possible that Black women who are in the early career stage may feel pressured to wear their hair straight or to wear certain types of clothing to "get their foot in the door."

Also, there is some research that points to Black women in leadership positions and senior career status may also engage in shifting. McDowell and Carter-Francique (2017) explored the experiences of African American female athletic directors and found that they discussed shifting or role flexing by shifting their behaviors or guarding their cultural behaviors when interacting with white people to avoid experiencing gendered racism (Jones and Shorter-Gooden 2003; Shorter-Gooden 2004). Similarly, Holder et al. (2012) found that Black women in senior-level positions working in corporate America discussed being challenged on their intellect, competence, and authority, and engaged in religion, shifting, and self-care as coping strategies.

STRESS ASSOCIATED WITH IDENTITY SHIFTING FOR BLACK WOMEN

The pain and frustration associated with experiences of gendered racial oppression, among other marginalized identities, remains a constant barrier to the survival of Black women in ivory communities, such as the workplace (Harris, 2007). In the workplace, there are rules that dictate what is considered to be professional and the dos and don'ts for people of color, such as Black women. Scholars suggest that there are "feeling rules, socially shared norms that influence how people try to feel emotionally in given social interactions, in which employees are expected to adhere to these rules in the workplace" (Wingfield, 2010). It is possible that a grasp of the mechanisms associated with identity shifting can assist with the understanding and potential prevention of major health concerns facing Black women.

Thus, the art of identity shifting can take a toll on Black women's physical and mental health, where they may feel prepared to alter their actions and appearance. Due to altering of Black women's speech, appearance, and perspectives, if there are any identity/self-concept discrepancies among Black women, then this can lead to anxiety and confusion, further affecting mental health (e.g., Higgins, 1987). Past studies have shown that while there are some benefits to engaging in identity shifting for Black women, it may come at a cost. For instance, Jones and colleagues (2021) found that greater involvement in identity shifting strategies was also positively correlated with higher levels of both depression symptoms and anxiety symptoms. In all, it can be psychologically taxing to shift one's language, appearance, and perspective in the workplace for Black women. This could leave other health implications such as burnout and psychological well-being.

Moreover, researchers have argued and illustrated that race-related stress, racial interactions between individuals or groups due to racism, is perceived to threaten one's well-being (Harrell, 2000). Studies have also shown that race-related stress is associated with decreased psychological and spiritual well-being; and, psychological functioning (Harrell, 2000). I would argue that due to gendered race-related stress, individual and group interactions due to racism and sexism that cause negative health outcomes have compounded for Black women and may cause even more adverse outcomes to their health. Past studies have shown the link between race-related stress and hypertension, blood pressure, obesity, diabetes, and cardiovascular disease (Cozier et al., 2016; Dolezsar et al., 2014; Hall et al., 2012). Similarly, to research on acculturation stress among immigrants, it can be argued that people of color, in particular Black women, may also experience stress when they engage in code-switching (Cross et al., 2017). In addition, Gamst and colleagues (2020) examined shifting, acculturation, and perceived race-related stress among Black women and found that immersion in the African American culture increased engagement in shifting behaviors and race-related stress. Past studies have shown that, "the need to portray an image of survival and strength prevents Black women from expressing their inner desires and needs, psychological distress, and depressive or anxiety symptoms" (Thomas et al., 2004, p. 430). Overall, engaging in identity shifting is exhausting and thus influences the psychological and physical health of Black women and can affect workplace dynamics by compromising the ability to form meaningful authentic relationships.

Based on this research suggesting the stress associated with identity shifting among Black women (Gamst et al., 2020; Jones et al., 2021), these results have implications for Black women scholars, activists, and clinicians. While there may remain a pressure to engage in identity shifting for some Black women in work or social settings to advance in their careers or enhance relationships, it is important to find a balance with shifting. The stress and other mental health costs that may come with engaging in shifting is due to the pressure and mixed feelings associated with not being able to be one's true self across different settings. As such, researchers should explore longitudinally the influence of shifting among Black women on other health outcomes, such as cardiovascular disease and trauma. There is research suggesting that there are benefits to authenticity, especially in the workplace, such as work and life satisfaction, formation of meaningful relationships, and more career opportunities (Dickens & Womack, 2020; Smith, 2008). However, it is important to not forget that being authentic in the workplace will not solve all the problems. While there are known benefits to authenticity in the workplace, it can also come at a cost for Black women. For some Black women who may choose to be more of their authentic self at work, it could cost them their job or respect by their colleagues. Though there are challenges with authenticity in the workplace for Black women, the benefits of shifting may outweigh the costs (Dickens & Womack, 2020). This work speaks to the costs to Black women's health due to engaging in identity shifting and the importance of choosing authenticity to promote one's wellness.

REFERENCES

Cozier, Y. C., Albert, M. A., Castro-Webb, N., Coogan, P. F., Ridker, P., Kaufman, H. W., ... Rosenberg, L. (2016). Neighborhood socioeconomic status in relation to serum biomarkers in the Black Women's Health Study. *Journal of Urban Health*, *93*(2), 279–291.

Cross, W. E., Jr., Seaton, E. K., Yip, T., Lee, R. M., Rivas, D., Gee, G. C., … Ngo, B. (2017). Identity work: Enactment of racial-ethnic identity in everyday life. http://doi.org/10.14288/1.0368597

Dickens, D. D., & Chavez, E. L. (2018). Navigating the workplace: The costs and benefits of shifting identities at work among early career us black women. *Sex Roles*, *78*(11–12), 760–774. https://doi.org/10.1007/s11199-017-0844-x
Dickens, D. D., & Womack, V. Y. (2020). Unapologetic authentic early career Black women: Challenging the dominant narrative. In Thomas K. M. (Ed.), *Diversity resistance in organizations* (pp. 21–33). Routledge.
Dickens, D. D., Womack, V. Y., & Dimes, T. (2019). Managing hypervisibility: An exploration of theory and research on identity shifting strategies in the workplace among Black women. *Journal of Vocational Behavior*, *113*, 153–163.
Dolezsar, C. M., McGrath, J. J., Herzig, A. J., & Miller, S. B. (2014). Perceived racial discrimination and hypertension: A comprehensive systematic review. *Health Psychology*, *33*(1), 20.
Fowler. (2021). Black woman fired for wearing natural hair instead of a wig, Louisiana lawsuit says. https://www.sunherald.com/news/nationworld/national/article255362471.html#storylink=cy
Gamst, G., Arellano-Morales, L., Meyers, L. S., Serpas, D. G., Balla, J., Diaz, A., ... Aldape, R. (2020). Shifting can be stressful for African American women: A structural mediation model. *Journal of Black Psychology*, *46*(5), 364–387.
Hall, J. C., Everett, J. E., & Hamilton-Mason, J. (2012). Black women talk about workplace stress and how they cope. *Journal of Black Studies*, *43*(2), 207–226.
Harrell, S. P. (2000). A multidimensional conceptualization of racism-related stress: Implications for the well-being of people of color. *American Journal of Orthopsychiatry*, *70*(1), 42–57.
Harrison, M. S. (2010). Colorism: The often un-discussed-ism in America's workforce. *Jury Expert*, *22*, 67.
Hill, M. E. (2002). Skin color and the perception of attractiveness among African Americans: Does gender make a difference? *Social Psychology Quarterly*, *65*(1), 77–91. https://doi.org/10.2307/3090169
Hunter, M. (2007). The persistent problem of colorism: Skin tone, status, and inequality. *Sociology Compass*, *1*(1), 237–254.
Jones, M. K., & Day, S. X. (2018). An exploration of Black women's gendered racial identity using a multidimensional and intersectional approach. *Sex Roles*, *79*(1–2), 1–15. https://doi.org/10.1007/s11199-017-0854-8
Jones, M. S., Womack, V., Jérémie-Brink, G., & Dickens, D. D. (2021). Gendered racism and mental health among young adult US Black women: The moderating roles of gendered racial identity centrality and identity shifting. *Sex Roles*, *85*(3), 221–231.
Jones, C., and Shorter-Gooden K. (2004). *Shifting: The double lives of African American women in America*. Darby, PA: Diane Publishing Company.
Lemi, D. C., & Brown, N. E. (2020). The political implications of colorism are gendered. *PS: Political Science & Politics*, *53*(4), 669–673.
Maddox, K. B., & Gray, S. A. (2002). Cognitive representations of Black Americans: Reexploring the role of skin tone. *Personality and Social Psychology Bulletin*, *28*(2), 250–259.

McDowell, J., & Carter-Francique, A. (2017). An intersectional analysis of the workplace experiences of African American female athletic directors. *Sex Roles*, *77*(5), 393–408.

Opie, T. R., & Phillips, K. W. (2015). Hair penalties: The negative influence of Afrocentric hair on ratings of Black women's dominance and professionalism. *Frontiers in Psychology*, *6*, 1311.

Smith, Y. (2008). Womanist theology: Empowering black women through Christian education. *Black Theology*, *6*(2), 200–220.

Thomas, A. J., Witherspoon, K. M., & Speight, S. L. (2004). Toward the development of the stereotypic roles for Black women scale. *Journal of Black Psychology*, *30*(3), 426–442.

Thomas, K. M., Johnson-Bailey, J., Phelps, R. E., Tran, N. M., & Johnson, L. (2013). Women of color at midcareer: Going from pet to threat. In L. Comas-Diaz & B. Green (Eds.), *The psychological health of women of color: Intersections, challenges, and opportunities* (pp. 275–286). Guilford Press.

Watson, L. B., Lewis, J. A., & Moody, A. T. (2019). A sociocultural examination of body image among Black women. *Body Image*, *31*, 280–287.

Wingfield, A. H. (2010). Are some emotions marked "whites only"? Racialized feeling rules in professional workplaces. *Social Problems*, *57*(2), 251–268.

Chapter 11

Eluding the White Gaze

Sex Education for Black Girls by Black Women

Sara C. Flowers

INTRODUCTION

Since[1] one of the first ships carrying enslaved people crested over the horizon toward the coast of Virginia in 1619, Black women have been creating, adapting, and evolving their sociocultural understanding of themselves, and their environment, through an intersectional framework[2] in order to survive in the Americas (Kendi, 2019; Kendall, 2021; Hill Collins, 1986, S14–32; Crenshaw, 1991, 1241–1299; Smith, 2019). This chapter will describe the way Black women sex educators have attempted to neutralize the impact of the white gaze by identifying erasure and interrupting patterns that reinforce harmful practices and stereotypes, in the manner that our foremothers taught us, in order to prioritize wellness, joy, wholeness, and hope. Black women sex educators recenter sex education in practice, with Black community and identity at the core, so that the Black girls they teach cannot just do more than survive, but they thrive.

The White Gaze, Defined

Renowned American novelist Toni Morrison coined the phrase *white gaze* to describe the way that white ethnocentrism asserts itself as the default context and narrative for the so-called "valid" cultural experiences throughout society (Assare, 2021; Greenfield-Sanders, 2020). The white gaze centers the white experience as the baseline from which all other activities are defined and assessed (Pitchford & Holtz, 2020; Smith, 2019). It presumes a white audience, and centers a white, cisgender, heterosexual, masculine lens. White ethnocentricity is the driving force behind the white gaze, positing that whiteness deserves to be the central tenant and vantage point of every story, experience, approach, and appraisal (Pitchford & Holtz, 2020). Unsurprisingly, in the United States, whiteness is often the lens through which literature, art, education, medicine, psychology, public health research and practice, and so much more are created, critiqued, operationalized, and evaluated (Bassett & Graves, 2018, 457–458; Assare, 2021; Greenfield-Sanders, 2020; Smith, 2019; Pitchford & Holtz, 2020).

White Ethnocentricity Is a Form of Structural Racism

Zinzi D. Bailey and colleagues define structural racism as ". . .the totality of ways in which societies foster racial discrimination through mutually reinforcing systems of housing, education, employment, earnings, benefits, credit, media, health care, and criminal justice" (2017). Leading Black scholars who study Black women and sexual health agree, stating that structural racism demonstrates ". . .a differential reduction of access . . . due to social structures and policies" and these effects impact the sexual health and well-being of Black women, and girls (Gilbert, 2021; Thompson et al., 2022, 195–202). It is no surprise then that white ethnocentricity is inextricably embedded in the American experience, including throughout the public health and education systems (Bailey et al., 2017, 1453–1463; Pitchford & Holtz, 2020; Sue, 2004, 761–769). According to these definitions, along with the exhaustive literature highlighting its presence and lasting impact in the United States for over 400 years, white ethnocentricity should be explicitly recognized as one of the many vehicles of structural racism.

Because forms of structural racism ". . . reinforce discriminatory beliefs, values, and distribution of resources" (Bailey et al., 2017, 1453–1463), no discipline within the social sciences is exempt from its ramifications. In the case of sex education, many sex education programs were likely developed for a Black youth audience without incorporating and centering the professional expertise, sociocultural understanding, and intersectional lens of Black sex educators (Opara et al., 2021, 12088; Laureano & Flowers, 2018, 50–60; Flowers, 2016; Gilbert, 2021; Floyd & Gary-Smith, n.d.). Furthermore, research used to underpin programs for Black girls largely utilize deficit frameworks when planning and developing curricula goals (Opara et al., 2021, 12088; Anderson, 2020, 86–100; Floyd & Gary-Smith, n.d.). This deficits-centric approach creates less effective and potentially harmful programs because critical socio-cultural factors, expertise, and community strengths, capacities, and context were omitted from the programs' development, design, implementation, and evaluation.

Context Matters

While data describing sexual and reproductive health disparities experienced by Black women, and girls are incontrovertible when compared to experiences of their white peers, both the data, and the Black women's, and girls' contextualized experiences themselves, deserve a more complex analysis of the circumstances through which the data were collected and analyzed, including the impact of systemic racism, cultural differences, and subconscious white ethnocentrism (Sue, 2004, 761–769; Thompson et al., 2022, 195–202; Gilbert, 2021; Prather et al., 2018, 249–259).

When public health data, stratified by race and gender, suggest sexual and reproductive health behavior and outcomes, the enduring presence of the white savior complex,[3] misogynoir,[4] and medical, institutional, and structural racism cannot be ignored (Prather et al., 2018, 249–259). Just because these influences may not explicitly be listed as confounding factors in program design and evaluation for sex education curricula targeting Black girls, their influence should not remain unconsidered, nor should we assume their effect is neutral or benign. In other words, (how) have program designers intentionally controlled for sociodemographic confounders in program development and delivery, especially when, due to racism, these particular confounding factors can only be experienced by Black program participants (Guan, 2021)? Examples of these racism-related confounding factors might include the individual curriculum author's or program evaluator's biases (conscious or unconscious). The presence of the white gaze and white ethnocentricity is embedded throughout the structure of the field, and therefore are also present in the product, pathways, and end-result-desired when analyzing these programs' fidelity and evaluation data.

Let's consider how [the presence of] the white gaze shaped the existence and evolution of sex education program development, sex educator training, and program evaluation. If the presence of white ethnocentricism and the white gaze is understood and irrefutable, it stands to reason that the field of sex education and its programs (development, facilitator training, program delivery, and program evaluation) were not immune from their effects (Floyd & Gary-Smith, n.d.).

In the United States, the profession of teaching is undervalued and underappreciated. Teachers and professors are neither paid in accordance with the responsibility they shoulder or the credentials they hold, nor is their expertise in pedagogy and human development as well respected as is deserved (Bruno, 2018). Similar to how teachers and professors specialize in particular subjects like history or math, sex educators' specific subject matter expertise is in the field of sex and sexuality; they integrate knowledge of sex, sexuality, and human development using pedagogical approaches and facilitation skills to help their students acquire multifaceted knowledge and skills that are applicable through the lifespan (Fields, 2008). Sex education provides learners with the foundational understanding that is needed to build and maintain healthy relationships with ourselves and with others (Johnson, 2018).

Sex educators encounter some of the same challenges and false assumptions that teachers and professors face, including being consistently underpaid and underappreciated, and having their professional expertise undervalued (i.e., the assumption that because sex is involved, it's easy and anyone can do it). To further complicate matters, sex educators also are frequently stereotyped as being hypersexual; some people have difficulty making sense of our comfort, deep knowledge, and familiarity with information that is typically shrouded in secrecy and shame. Misogynoir and the intersectional identities that Black sex educators hold compound the ways that these stereotypes negatively impact both individual sex educators and the field as "professional" more broadly.

Audre Lorde teaches us that there is power in the erotic (2007). She defines the erotic as going beyond sexual pleasure, to encompass the deep joy and fulfillment that we find in meaningful friendships, music, and creative outlets (Lorde, 2007; Fields, 2008). An investment in sex education is an investment in individual agency. It harbors the potential for learners to practice understanding and exploring new ideas, challenge existing structures, and invest in personal joy and wellness for oneself, and with others (Floyd & Gary-Smith, n.d.; Fields, 2008). Sex education builds community; sex educators cultivate learning spaces built on trust, safety, and mutual respect (Flowers et al., 2022, 87–105).

In her research, Jessica Fields notes that Black students were more likely than their white peers to receive warnings and risk advisories in sex education classes (2008). Only the affluent white students were encouraged to explore during adolescence; Black students and poor white students were warned about becoming teen parents and being diagnosed with sexually transmitted infections (Fields, 2008). In contrast, Black women sex educators see these inequalities in program design and delivery, and work to upend them. They recognize that Black youth deserve to grow up protected; they too should be invited to explore, and center their joy and humanity.

When Black women, and girls begin to understand the true and deep extent to which they are capable of finding joy, pleasure, and fulfillment—they inherently become part of the resistance, using their power to fight racism, sexism, and the patriarchy (Lorde, 2007). Black women sex educators know that when they create, nurture, and protect space to facilitate sex education curricula beyond the white gaze, they are making it possible for Black girls to learn to question, challenge, explore, and develop their agency safely.

The white gaze perpetuated long-standing negative stereotypes about Black girls that originated from systemic oppression, slavery, and racism, such as hypersexuality, high pain tolerance, and deriving pleasure from caring for others (specifically male partners, biological children, or children for whom they are caregivers) (Shaw & Shaw Nevins, 2006; Gilbert, 2021; Flowers, 2018, 308–325; Prather et al., 2018, 249–259; Opara et al., 2021, 12088). Historically, sexual health prevention programming sought to disrupt stigmatized sexual health outcomes that are disproportionately experienced by Black women, and girls by intervening at the individual level. This approach neglected to account for social determinants of health, including social, economic, and environmental factors (Opara et al., 2021, 12088; Thompson et al., 2022, 195–202; Fields, 2008). The impact of unintended pregnancy, sexually transmitted infections including HIV, and limited access to contraception, sex education, and accessible, affordable, inclusive culturally responsive healthcare is compounded by the centuries of racist policies and practices that set the foundation for Black women and girls sexual and reproductive health and well-being in the United States (Opara et al., 2021, 12088; Prather et al., 2018, 249–259).

Evidence-based interventions that were developed under the veil of the white gaze underestimated the ways that systems of oppression contributed to establishing and maintaining disparate outcomes and experiences for Black girls and their sexual health (Prather et al., 2018, 249–259). At the individual and community levels, Black women and girls were not set up for success when program interventions ignored or underestimated the gravitational pull that institutional, medical, and situational racism have on Black women/girls' sexual and reproductive health (Opara et al., 2021, 12088; Thompson et al., 2022, 195–202; Gilbert, 2021; Prather et al., 2018, 249–259). This underestimation inadvertently reinforced negative racial stereotypes that program developers presumably intended to eradicate (Prather et al., 2018, 249–259; Opara et al., 2021, 12088; Flowers, 2016). Black women sex educators created solutions for problems that they didn't cause; their ongoing love for and investment in their community and their hope for a better Black future are the catalysts that drive them to continue to center Black girls in their work (Flowers, 2016).

When systems of oppression are left unconsidered during the program/curriculum development stage, the effect of those omissions is not neutral. It follows that the decision to prioritize a deficits framework when developing sex education interventions for Black girls omitted and overlooked key protective factors that are unique to Black girls, Black culture, and their membership in Black community (Opara et al., 2021, 12088; Floyd & Gary-Smith, n.d.). For example, research exploring how race and gender differences impact self-esteem showed that adolescent Black girls whose scores demonstrated high levels of racial pride also had high scores in self-esteem and self-concept (Anderson, 2020, 86–100). Furthermore, ". . .adolescent Black girls often possess higher self-esteem when compared with other racial and ethnic groups . . ." including their white female peers (Anderson, 2020, 86–100). By definition, a deficits framework neglects to consider the ways that high self-esteem in Black girls might influence sexual health decisions positively; in contrast, adolescent Black girls' high self-esteem is an asset, which likely bolsters agency, joy, and wellness for those whose sex education is offered via a body-positive, sex-positive, pleasure-positive approach. From a data collection standpoint, needs assessments alone, which by definition only focus on deficits, are insufficient (Adamson, 2013). First, who defined what the deficits were? If an intended audience is not included, then once again, we find ourselves faced with the dynamic where outsiders assign value to an audience's qualities and experience using a vantage point and criteria that are externally driven and defined (Coreil, 2010, 274). White ethnocentricity is an assumed influence if and when mainstream (white) curriculum developers assign value for the Black intended audience without seeking input from Black community members and leaders.

> When we think about data, and how it's been gathered, is that, from marginalized communities, it was never gathered to help or serve us. It was primarily done to show the deficits in our communities, to show where there are gaps. And it's always done from a deficit-based framework. They talk about how our communities have the highest rates of obesity, have the highest rates of diabetes, highest rates of infant mortality. How our people may be experiencing high rates of opiate misuse.
>
> What they don't talk about is the strengths of our community . . . And so we were always strength-based people, who passed on and continued knowledge systems regardless of people who tried to destroy us (Abigail Echo-Hawk, Secaira & Sillman, 2019).

Alternatively, a community-centered, community-driven assessment that asks the community members themselves to define strengths and capacities, along with needs, will provide a more comprehensive lens of all of the dynamics that contribute to and influence Black girls' sexual health, including sex education, sexual behavior, healthcare access, and sexual health outcomes (Flowers et al., 2022, 87–105) (Coreil, 2010, 274) (Opara et al., 2021, 12088) (Gilbert, 2021).

WE KNOW THE SOLUTIONS WE NEED

According to Brittany N. Anderson, Black girls benefit from curricula and learning environments that value and reflect their backgrounds and community; she specifically names the ways that the intersectional approaches and Anti-Racist Pedagogy[5] support Black girls' learning and development (2020).

Black women sex educators leverage their multidimensional power when they utilize an intersectional sexuality education framework to develop, adapt, and deliver sex education programming for Black girls (Flowers, 2018, 308–325; Flowers, 2016). The model below illustrates the concurrent, iterative frameworks and processes that Black women sex educators use to facilitate, ". . .adapt, and tailor mainstream sex education curricula to meet the evolving needs of their intended audience" (Flowers, 2018, 308–325).

Theory-practice dyads are the central components of the Multidimensional Power framework (figure 11.1). They work together to describe the concurrent knowledge and skills application that Black women sex educators understand, adopt, and employ in service of their intended audience. According to *Enacting Our Multidimensional Power* (Flowers, 2018, 313–316), the Multidimensional Power framework theory-practice dyads include:

SOCIOCULTURAL UNDERSTANDING and BLACK FEMINIST THOUGHT

The shared, interlocking, historical experiences of oppression, self-definition, self-valuation, and cultural understanding identified and described through Black feminist thought uniquely positions Black women sex educators to combine their personal experiences with their professional knowledge and expertise in sexuality education to build a meaningful, relevant, experience-based rapport with their intended audience (particularly Black girls) (Hill Collins, 1986, S14–32).

PROFESSIONAL EXPERIENCE and THEORY OF GENDER AND POWER

The relationship between gender and power imbalances in society, heightened risk of sexually transmitted infections, and sexual inequality is well documented (Wingood and DiClemente, 2000; Peragallo et al., 2005; Dworkin et al., 2008; Tillman, 2002; Card, Solomon, and Cunningham, 2011). Black women experience these imbalances and integrate the knowledge gained from navigating social, economic, cultural, gendered, and race-based inequities with their professional expertise as sexual health educators to help students develop necessary coping skills, to offering empathy and support, or to suggest practical solutions based on lessons learned (Wingood and DiClemente, 2000; Gómez, 2011). It follows that knowledge and skills acquired by young Black women participants in sex education programs facilitated by Black women sex educators may relate to sociocultural topics specific to the lived experiences of women of color that

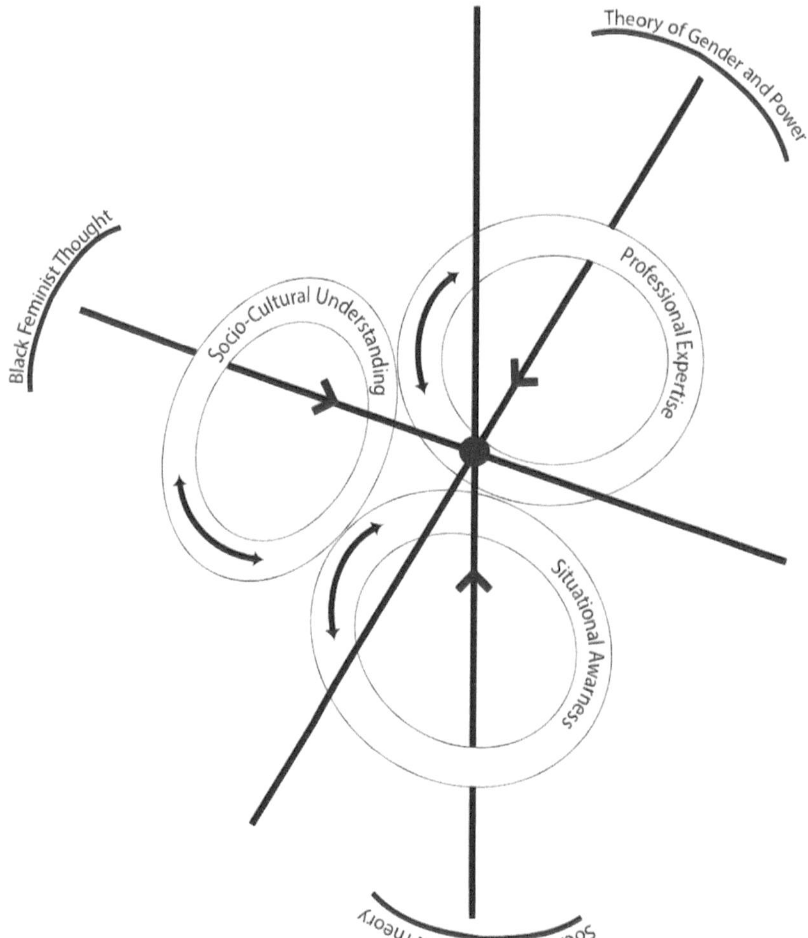

Figure 11.1 Multidimensional Power: An Intersectional Sexuality Education Model (Flowers, 2016; Flowers, 2018, 308-325). *Source*: Created by author.

are otherwise not explicitly articulated in sex education curricula (Flowers, 2016).

SITUATIONAL AWARENESS and SOCIAL CONSTRUCTIVIST THEORY

Social constructivist theory recognizes that learners contribute to the development and acquisition of knowledge in sex education classes and workshops, and that interactive learning is a key method to developing new knowledge, skills, and abilities (Mallory and New, 1994). When implementing sex education curricula with Black girls, learning about sexuality, gender norms, and relationships, for example, is often framed by participants' social environment, culture,

> religion, gender identity, and sexual orientation (Prather et al., 2016). Black women sex educators have a mutual understanding of ways in which sociocultural experiences influence learners' acquisition of knowledge, skills, and abilities, and they use that mutual understanding to provide relevant examples, adapt curricula to ensure that lessons and discussions are culturally congruent, and, in turn, strengthen the learning that that is taking place during a sex education class or workshop. (Carroll et al., 2007)

Black girls benefit from the ways that Black women sex educators operationalize the Mutltidemensional Power framework to deliver representative sex education. Research shows that representation in learning matters (Future of Sex Education Initiative, 2020; Flowers, 2018, 308–325; Day et al., 2019, 29–43; Floyd & Gary-Smith, n.d.). This is true in most any subject—including history, social studies, literature—and yep, sex education too! All students benefit when they see their lived experiences, and that of their classmates and community members, reflected in the people and stories featured in literature and history books (Day et al., 2019, 29–43). With respect to Black girls and sex education, this phenomenon holds true (Flowers et al., 2022, 87–105; Future of Sex Education Initiative, 2020). When Black girls don't see their lives and experiences reflected in sex education curriculum or content, or if the way they are represented is tokenizing, rooted in stereotypes and racist tropes instead of reality, the erasure and misrepresentation creates a disconnect between the content and the learner (Advocates for Youth, 2015; Flowers, 2016; Future of Sex Education Initiative, 2020; Anderson, 2020, 86–100). As a result of this disconnect, it may be challenging for Black girls to relate to the lessons, and in turn, find it difficult to apply those lessons to their own lives (Advocates for Youth, 2015; Flowers, 2016; Future of Sex Education Initiative, 2020).

There is an abundance of literature by Black scholars that identify and describe phenomena that uphold white supremacy in institutions, and also outline how to eradicate it. It is impossible to include an exhaustive list of examples in this chapter; however a shortlist of key thought leaders and their contributions must be named. In 1986, Patricia Hill Collins described the phenomenon known as Black Feminist Thought (Hill Collins, 1986, S14–32). In 1989, Kimberlé Crenshaw offered the framework of intersectionality to the world (Crenshaw, 1989, 139–167; Crenshaw, 1991, 1241–1299). In 1995, critical race theorists, most of whom are scholars of color, assembled and published a body of literature and scholarly thinking that clearly articulates not only the plethora of interconnected ways that white supremacy operates in the relationship between society and the law in the United States, but also seeks to go beyond understanding that relationship's existence, to proposing ways to change it (Peller et al., 1995); In 2019, Nikole Hannah-Jones spearheaded the game-changing anthology known as *The 1619 Project*, shifting the foundational understanding of the history of the United States and its inextricable relationship with slavery (Smith, 2019). In 2020, Mikki Kendall offered a previously unconsidered description of issues central to Black womanhood and femininity in *Hood Feminism: Notes From The Women That A Movement Forgot* (Kendall, 2021).

What's incredible about the short list of scholarly contributions named above is how frequently, repeatedly, and often with vehemence, the concepts within are ignored, disregarded, dismissed, or outright attacked (Serwer, 2019; Strauss & Rockman, 2021; Sawchuk, 2021; Coaston, 2019).

And, the attacks continue. In this notably egregious, but unfortunately, not unprecedented moment in history—when literature written by and centering the true stories of Black, Indigenous, and other people of color are continually being banned from schools and libraries, we find ourselves once again faced with the narrative that our lived experience threatens the self-aggrandized white, cisgender, heteronormative, masculine agenda, and so must be eradicated, under the guise of our reality being invalid and threatening to white ethnocentrism (Sarappo, 2021; Sarappo, 2022; Strauss, 2022; Pitchford & Holtz, 2020).

Common themes that many of the banned books share is that the narrative describes the (sometimes harsh) realities that people/characters experience(d) due to the intersectional identities they hold (Strauss, 2022). In some circumstances, banned books depict the way racism, homophobia, transphobia, misogyny, misogynoir, ableism, anti-semitism, and other systems of oppression are pervasive in American history and current events, and the way that those experiences are inextricable from life as a whole (Sarappo, 2021). In others, the main character is simply not white (Good Reads, 2021). In both instances, censoring the complexity of the human experience through the white gaze harms individuals and society as a whole; but erasure is specifically notable, and harmful, to the people whose experiences are invalidated by that erasure (Anderson, 2020, 86–100).

Subjective and incomplete truths, along with an insistence on referencing a one-sided perspective, are irresponsible, short-sighted, and harmful. The best programming ideally includes an accurate and complete set of facts, and panoramic perspective as a foundation. We know Blackness, or Black race, in and of itself is not a risk factor for health disparities. But Black people, who live their entire lives in a system built and maintained by white supremacy, are vulnerable to health disparities because of the way they are affected by racism. "Structural racism affects both population and individual health in three interrelated domains: redlining and racialized residential segregation, mass incarceration and police violence, and unequal medical care" (Bailey et al., 2021, 768–773). Racist values that have been integrated throughout our society for centuries without question have led to Black people being perceived as less human, and ultimately less deserving of empathy (Washington, 2008). Lack of empathy then reinforces the justification, rationalization, or dismissal of unjust policies and treatment that Black folks navigate while trying to survive under the confines of structural racism.

BLACK SEX EDUCATORS ARE MAGIC

Black women sex educators understand the negative impact erasure has on Black girls' learning, and are intentional about mitigating its impact by making adaptations that both meet curricula learning objectives and affirm Black girls' lived experiences (Flowers, 2016) (Anderson, 2020, 86–100). Similar to how Mikki Kendall (2021) shines a spotlight on issues that are central to women of color after they were ignored or overlooked by white feminism, Black sex educators identify the ways Black girls' lived experiences went unacknowledged and unconsidered in the development, publication, and evaluation of some evidence-based interventions (Flowers, 2016). After they identify the gaps that exist in some sex education curricula, Black women sex educators make adaptations so the pedagogy they employ is more inclusive and representative of the learners' lives—namely by applying and integrating anti-racist, intersectional, sex-positive frameworks in sex education program content that they are responsible for facilitating (Flowers, 2016; Flowers, 2018, 308–325; Future of Sex Education Initiative, 2020; Opara et al., 2021, 12088). These approaches are demonstrated to have a positive impact on Black girls' learning and sexual health outcomes (Opara et al., 2021, 12088; Anderson, 2020, 86–100).

There is a dearth of literature describing the ways Black women sex educators have honed their sociocultural understanding through an intersectional framework in service of centering Black girls' wellness and joy—and their approach denotes a marked shift away from the risk reductionist framework leveraged through and by the white gaze (Hill Collins, 1986, S14–32; Crenshaw, 1991, 1241–1299; Crenshaw, 1989, 139–167; Laureano & Flowers, 2018, 50–60; Flowers, 2016; Flowers, 2018, 308–325; Anderson, 2020, 86–100). This continuous cognitive process is done while simultaneously upholding the learning objectives and skills development that is core to sex education programming (Flowers, 2016).

Black women sex educators have gone on record to describe the various ways the curricula they implemented missed the mark with the programs' intended Black audiences (Flowers, 2016; Flowers, 2018, 308–325). Furthermore, they've been clear that leveraging their professional expertise, socio-cultural understanding, and situational awareness in order to make adaptations that strengthen the curriculum content and delivery is not universally well-received by powers that be. For example, grant administrators and funders often prioritized the value of program fidelity über alles—even when the students themselves found the content to be dated, culturally incongruent, offensive, and off-putting (Flowers, 2016).

To change this practice, and improve the experience and outcomes by and for Black girls, Black women sex educators understand that integrating the complex reality of our lived experience is central to our ability to thrive (Thompson et al., 2022, 195–202; Kendall, 2021; Flowers, 2018, 308–325; Flowers, 2016; Sex Education Collaborative, 2022; Anderson, 2020, 86–100; Opara et al., 2021, 12088). It follows that the presence and impact of these elements must be considered and calculated at each stage and phase in sex education program development and delivery, including: when defining an issue and priority audience, developing and delivering tailored programming/interventions, and evaluating the intended versus actual impact and outcomes of the intervention.

In my professional experience, both as a Black sex educator working with Black girls in Washington, DC and New York City from 2003 to 2018, and through research that I conducted with women of color sex educators, veteran Black women sex educators repeatedly described the ways the curricula they were charged with implementing lacked relevance for their intended audiences (Flowers et al., 2022, 87–105; Flowers, 2016; Flowers, 2018, 308–325; Gilbert, 2021). Young people complained about the overwhelmingly white characters and storylines as completely unrelatable (Flowers, 2016). Black women sex educators are intentional in the ways they work to strengthen and evolve sex education curricula, both overtly and covertly (Flowers, 2016). Some sought permission to supplement the supportive learning materials assigned to their curricula so that videos and content were more culturally congruent with that of their program participants; others created new content in order to help develop a new knowledge base or skill set (Flowers, 2016). All of these approaches put Black girls' physical, sexual, and emotional health and well-being at the center of the process, from design, to implementation, to evaluation (Flowers et al., 2022, 87–105). Black women sex educators steer Black girls away from a potentially stereotype-reinforcing risk reduction framework, and toward a more joy and wellness-centered approach that integrates our community's lived experiences with the knowledge and skills our children need to thrive (Flowers, 2016; Opara et al., 2021, 12088).

SEX EDUCATION EVOLUTION

The field of sex education integrates research and practice from many fields, with a particular focus on public health and pedagogy (Goldfarb & Lieberman, 2021, 13–27). In the United States, the institutions of education and public health—and so many others, including medicine—have long-standing/deep-rooted connections to research and academia—and white ethnocentrism pervades those fields as well (Konkel, 2015, A297–A302).

As the field of sex education continues to evolve, so too do the paradigms that guide our programs and practice. The approaches that were used to design and evaluate sex education programs helped establish the field's foundation through solid behavior change science were important, meaningful and imperfect; we as a field must grapple with these two truths. With the value and promise of sex education well established in the literature (Goldfarb & Lieberman, 2021, 13–27; Flowers et al., 2022, 87–105), there is an opportunity to ameliorate our original approaches, and respond to the active calls for improvement to strengthen our offerings for the next generation (Flowers, 2018, 308–325;Flowers, 2016; Ang Fonte, 2022; Future of Sex Education Initiative, 2020). Sex education leaders nationwide are calling for intersectional approaches to be embedded into sex education research and practice (Ang Fonte, 2022; Sex Education Collaborative, 2022; Flowers, 2018; Goldfarb & Lieberman, 2021, 13–27).

BLACK JOY IS A FORM OF RESISTANCE

One clear and often unnamed benefit of sex education is that Black women sex educators are intentional about centering Black girls' joy (Fields, 2008; Flowers, 2016; Flowers, 2018, 308–325). They operationalize this intention by adapting sex education curricula (formally or informally) that were originally drafted to address the problem with (presumedly hypersexual) Black girls, such as unintended teen pregnancy and STI transmission rates, which are in and of themselves sexual and reproductive health outcomes that were defined problematic by the white gaze (Flowers, 2016; Flowers, 2018, 308–325; Fields, 2008; Flowers et al., 2022, 87–105). When Black women sex educators go a step further by authoring new curricula and approaches that intentionally and unequivocally center Black girls from its inception, they are operationalizing the way Toni Morrison teachings by centering our Black experience and potential, eluding the white gaze. (Laureano & Flowers, 2018, 50–60; Gilbert, 2021).

Across the United States, Black women sex educators continue to change the game in service of Black girls. Without ownership or autonomy, our ancestors' bodies were used to establish the foundation of the field of sexual and reproductive health (Washington, 2008). Today, our leadership in this field firmly positions Black women as authors—subjects, no longer—of our sexual health, joy, and destiny. Below are non-exhaustive, non-mutually exclusive descriptions of just a few ways Black women sex educators are actively establishing a new foundation, in both policy and practice, for the evolving field of sex education:

Centering Accessibility and Learning in Community

> Thought leaders Bianca I. Laureano and Tracie Q. Gilbert are shifting the field by authoring curricula, conceptualizing frameworks that use a strengths-based approach to center Blackness in the intersection of race and sexuality, and by training new and seasoned sex educators to center communities of color, leverage justice frameworks to disrupt systems of oppression, and reclaim our humanity through liberation (Laureano, 2020) (Gilbert, 2021) (Laureano & Flowers, 2018, 50–60). Mariotta Gary-Smith, Cindy Lee Alves, Trina Scott, and Bianca I. Laureano created community for Black sex educators when they founded the Women of Color Sexual Health Network (WoCSHN), which exists to create opportunities for inclusion and retention of women/gender expansive folx of color in the Sexuality profession (including sexual science and Sexology); and intentionally challenges the white supremacy the field was built upon. (Women of Color Sexual Health Network, n.d.)

Center Body Positivity, Joy, Rest, and Pleasure

Black womensex educators and researchers intentionally center joy, rest, pleasure, and the beauty found in all bodies. They leverage their knowledge of sex, sexuality, and the beauty in Blackness to recharge our bodies and souls through podcasts and trainings (in-person and online). Dr. Lexx Brown James, a sex therapist and an educator, teaches and models sex positive parenting using the hashtag, #ShameFreeSexEd (Brown James, n.d.); Melissa Pintor Carnagey, founder and lead educator of Sex Positive Families, uses a shame-free, comprehensive, pleasure-positive approach to help parents raise sexually healthy children (Pintor Carnagey, n.d.).

Make no mistake—sex education is a distinct expertise. Black joy is resistance. Black womensex educators leverage their professional expertise and socio-cultural understanding to design and deliver intersectional sex education which in turn supports Black girls in their development, creating personal agency, bodily autonomy, and fostering joy. Black sex educators know that centering Black identity in their work nurtures our relationships with ourselves, others, and our community; it cultivates joy in our mission for liberation and justice; and it is proactively working to dismantle the systems that tried to steal our joy in the first (gottdamn!) place (Flowers, 2018, 308–325; Floyd & Gary-Smith, n.d.).

NOTES

1. The term *sex education* always refers to comprehensive sex education; abstinence-only-until-marriage or sexual risk avoidance (SRA) programming is not sex education and is not referenced here in any way.
2. Kimberlé Crenshaw coined the term intersectionality to describe seeing the ways that ". . .various forms of inequality often operate together and exacerbate each other" (Steinmetz, 2020).
3. White Savior Complex is a concept that originated in Western Imperialism, and driven by the underlying belief that a white person knows what's best for folks or communities who are Black, Indigenous, or other people of color, so that white person steps in, asserting their agenda and preferences to people of color, under the guise of lending assistance (Murphy, 2021).
4. Misogynoir is a term coined by Dr. Moya Bailey that describes the specific intersection of racism and sexism that is only experienced by Black women (Ruiz, 2020) (Retta & Bailey, 2021).
5. Anti-Racist Pedagogy is a Critical Theory paradigm that works to explain and counteract the persistence and impact of racism; this approach can be applied to any field of study (Chew et al., n.d.; Blakeney, 2005, 119–132).

REFERENCES

Adamson, L. (2013). *Girls Impact Aliquippa: A Community Health Capacity and Needs Assessment Proposal* [Master Essay]. University of Pittsburgh. http://d-scholarship.pitt.edu/19598/

Advocates for Youth. (2015, February 12). *A Call to Action: LGBTQ Youth Need Inclusive Sex Education*. Advocates for Youth. Retrieved March 7, 2022, from https://www.advocatesforyouth.org/posts/a-call-to-action-lgbtq-youth-need-inclusive-sex-education/

Anderson, B. N. (2020, March 18). "See Me, See Us": Understanding the Intersections and Continued Marginalization of Adolescent Gifted Black Girls in U.S. Classrooms. *Gifted Child Today*, *43*(2), 86–100. https://doi.org/10.1177%2F1076217519898216

Ang Fonte, J. (2022). *Comprehensive Means Intersectional: Moving Sex Education Forward* [Keynote Address]. Amaze. https://youtu.be/RaTpGuZbToI

Assare, J. G. (2021, December 28). *Understanding The White Gaze And How It Impacts Your Workplace*. forbes.com. Retrieved March 3, 2022, from https://www.forbes.com/sites/janicegassam/2021/12/28/understanding-the-white-gaze-and-how-it-impacts-your-workplace/?sh=466a5b154cd6

Bailey, Z. D., Feldman, J. M., & Bassett, M. T. (2021, February 25). How Structural Racism Works—Racist Policies as a Root Cause of U.S. Racial Health Inequalities.

The New England Journal of Medicine, *384*(8), 768–773. https://www.nejm.org/doi/full/10.1056/NEJMms2025396

Bailey, Z. D., Krieger, N., Agénor, M., Graves, J., Linos, N., & Bassett, M. T. (2017, April 08). Structural Racism and Health Inequities in the USA: Evidence and Interventions. *The Lancet*, *389*(10077), 1453–1463. https://doi.org/10.1016/S0140-6736(17)30569-X

Bassett, M. T., & Graves, J. D. (2018). Uprooting Institutionalized Racism as Public Health Practice. *American Journal of Public Health*, *108*(4), 457–458. 10.2105/AJPH.2018.304314

Blakeney, A. M. (2005). Antiracist Pedagogy: Definition, Theory, and Professional Development. *Journal of Curriculum and Pedagogy*, *2*(1), 119–132.

Brown James, L. (n.d.). *Shame Free Sex Ed.* Dr. Lexx, The Sex Doc. Retrieved March 9, 2022, from https://www.lexxsexdoc.com/for sexed4dads

Bruno, R. (2018, June 20). When Did the US Stop Seeing Teachers as Professionals? *Harvard Business Review*. Retrieved March 10, 2022, from https://hbr.org/2018/06/when-did-the-u-s-stop-seeing-teachers-as-professionals

Card, J. J., Solomon, J., & Cunningham, S. D. (2011, January). How to Adapt Effective Programs for Use in New Contexts. *Health Promotion Practice*, *12*(1), 25–35. https://doi.org/10.1177/1524839909348592

Carroll, C., Patterson, M., Wood, S., Booth, A., Rick, J., & Balain, S. (2007, November). A Conceptual Framework for Implementation Fidelity. *Implementation Science*, *2*(40), 1–9. https://doi.org/10.1186/1748-5908-2-40

Chew, S., Houston, A., Cooper, A., & Glasper, R. (n.d.). *An Introductory Guide to Building an Anti-racist Pedagogy in Any Discipline Through Instructor Reflection, Clear Communication g*. UNC Gillings School of Global Public Health. Retrieved March 9, 2022, from https://sph.unc.edu/wp-content/uploads/sites/112/2020/08/Anti_Racist_Discussion_Pedagogy__1.pdf

Coaston, J. (2019, May 28). *Intersectionality, Explained: Meet Kimberlé Crenshaw, Who Coined the Term*. Vox. Retrieved March 6, 2022, from https://www.vox.com/the-highlight/2019/5/20/18542843/intersectionality-conservatism-law-race-gender-discrimination

Collins, P. H. (2000). *Black Feminist Thought: Knowledge, Consciousness, and the Politics of Empowerment*. Routledge.

Coreil, J. (Ed.). (2010). *Social and Behavioral Foundations of Public Health*. SAGE Publications.

Crenshaw, K. (1989). Demarginalizing the Intersection of Race and Sex: A Black Feminist Critique of Antidiscrimination Doctrine, Feminist Theory and Antiracist Politics. *University of Chicago Legal Forum*, *1989*(1), 139–167. https://chicagounbound.uchicago.edu/cgi/viewcontent.cgi?article=1052&context=uclf

Crenshaw, K. (1991, July). Mapping the Margins: Intersectionality, Identity Politics, and Violence Against Women of Color. *Stanford Law Review*, *43*(6), 1241–1299. https://doi.org/doi.org/10.2307/1229039

Day, J. K., Ioverno, S., & Russell, S. T. (2019). Safe and Supportive Schools for LGBT Youth: Addressing Educational Inequities Through Inclusive Policies and Practices. *Journal of School Psychology*, *74*, 29–43.

Dworkin, S. L., Pinto, R. M., Hunter, J., Rapkin, B., & Remien, R. H. (2008, September). Keeping the Spirit of Community Partnerships alive in the Scale up of HIV/AIDS prevention: Critical Reflections on the Roll Out of DEBI (Diffusion of Effective Behavioral Interventions). *American Journal of Community Psychology, 42*(1–2), 51–59. https://doi.org/10.1007/s 10464-008-9183-y

Fields, J. (2008). *Risky Lessons: Sex Education and Social Inequality*. Rutgers University Press.

Flowers, S. C. (2016, September 30). Perceptions of Fidelity and Adaptation in Evidence-Informed Interventions by Women of color Sexuality Health Educators. In *Dissertations, Theses, and Capstone Projects*. CUNY Academic Works. https://academicworks.cuny.edu/gc_etds/1586/

Flowers, S. C. (2018). Enacting our Multidimensional Power: Black Women Sex Educators Demonstrate the Value of an Intersectional Framework. *Meridians: Feminism, Race, Transnationalism, 16*(2), 308–325. https://muse.jhu.edu/article/696143

Flowers, S. C., Krushnic, D., Levine, D., & Birnel Henderson, S. (2022). Sisterhood Unexpected: "I Met My Best Friend in LEAP!" and Other Narratives by LEAP for Girls Alumnae New York City, 2006–2016. In T. Bertrand J, S. Rahming, J. Andrews, & D. Davis Maye (Eds.), *Black Sisterhoods: Paradigms and Praxis* (pp. 87–105). Demeter Press.

Floyd, N., & Gary-Smith, M. (n.d.). *Sex Ed is a Vehicle for Racial Justice* [Interview]. SIECUS: Sex Ed for Social Change. https://siecus.org/sex-ed-is-a-vehicle-for-racial-justice/

Future of Sex Education Initiative. (2020). *National Sex Education Standards: Core Content and Skills, K-12* (2nd ed.). Future of Sex Education. https://afy1.wpengine.com/resources/health-information/future-of-sex-education-national-sexuality-education-standards/

Gilbert, T. Q. (n.d.). *The Sex Ed of Blackfolk*. TSOB--The Sex Ed of Blackfolk Podcast. Retrieved March 9, 2022, from https://www.tsobpodcast.com/

Gilbert, T. Q. (2021). Dr. Tracie Q. Gilbert. Retrieved March 9, 2022, from https://www.drtracieg.com/

Gilbert, T. Q. (2021). *Black and Sexy: A Framework of Racialized Sexuality*. Taylor & Francis Limited.

Goldfarb, E. S., & Lieberman, L. D. (2021). Three Decades of Research: The Case for Comprehensive Sex Education. *Journal of Adolescent Health, 68*, 13–27. https://doi.org/10.1016/j.jadohealth.2020.07.036

Gómez, C. A. (2011, November–December). Preventing HIV in U.S. Women and Girls: A Call for Social Action. *Women's Health Issues, 21*(6), S287–S294. https://doi.org/10.1016/j.whi.2011.07.012

Good Reads. (2021, September 22). *Central York School District (2021) Banned Books List (299 books)*. Goodreads. Retrieved March 4, 2022, from https://www.goodreads.com/list/show/167218.Central_York_School_District_2021_Banned_Books_List

Greenfield-Sanders, T. (2020, June 22). Toni Morrison on Writing Without the "White Gaze" | American Masters. *PBS*. https://www.pbs.org/wnet/americanmasters/toni-morrison-on-writing-without-the-white-gaze/14874/

Guan, M. (2021, November 29). Sexual and Reproductive Health Knowledge, Sexual Attitudes, and Sexual Behaviour of University Students: Findings of a Beijing-Based Survey in 2010–2011. *Archives of Public Health, 79*(215). https://doi.org/10.1186/s13690-021-00739-5

Hill Collins, P. (1986). Learning from the Outsider Within: The Sociological Significance of Black Feminist Thought. *Societal Problems, 33*(6), S14–32. doi.org/10.2307/800672.

An Interview with Dr. Bianca I. Laureano – DASAN. (2021, January). Pleasurable – Disability and Sexuality Education and Advocacy. Retrieved March 9, 2022, from https://dasanetwork.org/projects/podcast/dr-bianca-i-laureano/

Johnson, S. (2018). [Personal Communication]. In https://www.linkedin.com/in/shelagh-johnson/. Portland, OR.

Kendall, M. (2021). *Hood Feminism: Notes from the Women That a Movement Forgot.* Penguin Publishing Group.

Kendi, I. X. (2019, August 20). The Historical Significance of 1619. *The Atlantic.* https://www.theatlantic.com/ideas/archive/2019/08/historical-significance-1619/596365/

Konkel, L. (2015, December). Racial and Ethnic Disparities in Research Studies The Challenge of Creating More Diverse Cohorts. *Environmental Health Perspectives, 123*(12), A297–A302. https://www.ncbi.nlm.nih.gov/pmc/articles/PMC4670264/

Laureano, B. I. (2020). *About ANTE UP!* Ante Up! – Professional Development. Retrieved March 9, 2022, from https://www.anteuppd.com/our-team/

Laureano, B. I., & Flowers, S. C. (2018). Writing Ourselves Into Existence: Healing Through Collaborative Curriculum Development. *Journal of Critical Thought and Praxis, 7*(2), 50–60. https://dr.lib.iastate.edu/handle/20.500.12876/52455

Lorde, A. (2007). *Sister Outsider: Essays and Speeches (Crossing Press Feminist Series).* Crossing Press.

Mallory, B. L., & New, R. S. (1994, Fall). Social Constructivist Theory and Principles of Inclusion: Challenges for Early Childhood. *Journal of Special Education, 28*(3), 322–337.

Murphy, C. (2021, September 20). What Is White Savior Complex and Why Is It Harmful? | Health.com. *Health Magazine.* Retrieved March 9, 2022, from https://www.health.com/mind-body/health-diversity-inclusion/white-savior-complex

Opara, I., Abrams, J. A., Cross, K., & Amutah-Onukagha, N. (2021, November 18). Reframing Sexual Health for Black Girls and Women in HIV/STI Prevention Work: Highlighting the Role of Identity and Interpersonal Relationships. *International Journal of Environmental Research and Public Health, 18*(22), 12088. https:// doi.org/10.3390/ijerph182212088

Peller, G., Thomas, K., Crenshaw, K., & Gotanda, N. (Eds.). (1995). *Critical Race Theory: The Key Writings that Formed the Movement.* New Press.

Peragallo, N., DeForge, B., O'Campo, P., Lee, S. M., Kim, Y. J., Cianelli, R., & Ferrer, L. (2005, March–April). A Randomized Clinical Trial of an HIV-Risk-Reduction Intervention Among Low-Income Latina Women. *Nursing Research, 54*(2), 108-118.

Pintor Carnagey, M. (n.d.). *Sex Positive Families*. Sex Positive Families: Home. Retrieved March 9, 2022, from http://sexpositivefamilies.com

Pitchford, M., & Holtz, J. (2020, February 21). Beware of the White Gaze – Fourteen East. *14 East Magazine*. http://fourteeneastmag.com/index.php/2020/02/21/11505/

Prather, C., Fuller, T. R., Jeffries, IV, W. L., Marshall, K. J., Howell, A. V., Belyue-Umole, A., & King, W. (2018, September 22). Racism, African American Women, and Their Sexual and Reproductive Health: A Review of Historical and Contemporary Evidence and Implications for Health Equity. *Health Equity*, *2*(1), 249–259. http://doi.org/10.1089/heq.2017.0045

Prather, C., Fuller, T. R., Marshall, K. J., & Jeffries, W. J. (2016, July). The Impact of Racism on the Sexual and Reproductive Health of African American Women. *Journal of Women's Health*, *25*(7), 664–671. https:// doi.org/10.1089/jwh.2015.5637

Retta, M., & Bailey, M. (2021, May 19). *Moya Bailey's "Misogynoir Transformed" Breaks Down the Viral Term*. Bitch Media. Retrieved March 7, 2022, from https://www.bitchmedia.org/article/moya-bailey-misogynoir-transformed-interview

Ruiz, R. (2020, April 7). *4 Things You Need to Know About 'misogynoir'*. Mashable. Retrieved March 7, 2022, from https://mashable.com/article/misogynoir-black-women-sexism-racism

Sarappo, E. (2021, December 8). 10 Books Texas Officials Want to Ban From Schools. *The Atlantic*. https://www.theatlantic.com/culture/archive/2021/12/texas-book-ban-between-the-world-and-me/620938/

Sarappo, E. (2022, February 1). Book Bans Are Back. Here's What's In Danger. *The Atlantic*. https://www.theatlantic.com/books/archive/2022/02/banned-books-list-to-kill-a-mockingbird-maus/621428/

Sawchuk, S. (2021, May 18). *What Is Critical Race Theory, and Why Is It Under Attack?* Education Week. Retrieved March 6, 2022, from https://www.edweek.org/leadership/what-is-critical-race-theory-and-why-is-it-under-attack/2021/05

Secaira, M., & Sillman, M. (2019, May 31). *Abigail Echo-Hawk on the Art and Science of 'decolonizing Data'*. Crosscut. Retrieved March 10, 2022, from https://crosscut.com/2019/05/abigail-echo-hawk-art-and-science-decolonizing-data

Serwer, A. (2019, December 23). The Fight Over the 1619 Project Is Not About the Facts. *The Atlantic*. https://www.theatlantic.com/ideas/archive/2019/12/historians-clash-1619-project/604093/

Sex Education Collaborative. (2022, March). Comprehensive Means Intersectional: Moving Sex Education Forward. In *Resources*. Sex Education Collaborative. https://sexeducationcollaborative.org/comprehensive-means-intersectional

Shaw, A. E., & Shaw Nevins, A. (2006). *The Embodiment of Disobedience: Fat Black Women's Unruly Political Bodies*. Lexington Books.

Smith, C. (2019, August 14). The 1619 Project. *The New York Times*. https://www.nytimes.com/interactive/2019/08/14/magazine/1619-america-slavery.html

Smith, J. (2019, August 7). Toni Morrison: Author Helped Black People See Themselves in Stories. *Rolling Stone*. https://www.rollingstone.com/culture/culture-features/toni-morrison-author-beloved-tribute-868572/

Steinmetz, K. (2020, February 20). *Kimberlé Crenshaw on What Intersectionality Means Today | Time*. TIME. Retrieved March 10, 2022, from https://time.com/5786710/kimberle-crenshaw-intersectionality/

Strauss, V. (2022, February 10). Analysis | This Wave of Book Bans Is Different from Earlier Ones. *The Washington Post*. https://www.washingtonpost.com/education/2022/02/10/book-bans-maus-bluest-eye/

Strauss, V., & Rockman, S. (2021, April 7). Perspective | Why Republican Efforts to Ban the 1619 Project from Classrooms are so Misguided. *The Washington Post*. https://www.washingtonpost.com/education/2021/04/07/why-republican-efforts-to-ban-1619-project-classrooms-are-so-misguided/

Sue, D. W. (2004). Whiteness and Ethnocentric Monoculturalism: Making the "Invisible" Visible. *American Psychologist*, *59*(8), 761–769. https://doi.org/10.1037/0003-066X.59.8.761

Thompson, T. M., Young, Y.-Y., Bass, T. M., Baker, S., Njoku, O., Norwood, J., & Simpson, M. (2022, February). Racism Runs Through It: Examining the Sexual and Reproductive Health Experience of Black Women in the South. *Health Affairs*, *41*(2), 195–202. 10.1377/hlthaff.2021.01422

Tillman, L. C. (2010). I'm No Jezebel; I Am Young, Gifted, and Black: Identity, Sexuality, and Black Girls. *Psychology of Women Quarterly*, *34*(3), 273–285. https://doi.org/10.1111/j.1471-6402.2010.01574.x

Washington, H. A. (2008). *Medical Apartheid: The Dark History of Medical Experimentation on Black Americans from Colonial Times to the Present*. Harlem Moon.

Wingood, G. M., & DiClemente, R. J. (2000, October). Application of the Theory of Gender and Power to Examine HIV-Related Exposures, Risk Factors, and Effective Interventions for Women. *Health Education & Behavior*, *27*(5), 539–565. https://doi.org/10.1177/109019810002700502

Women of Color Sexual Health Network. (n.d.). WoCSHN. Retrieved March 9, 2022, from http://wocshn.org

Chapter 12

Black Women Stay Fighting Structural Racism

Other-mothering as Community Praxis

Maranda Ward

PHILOSOPHY OF SCIENCE

My mom was the matriarch of my nuclear and extended family.[1] She witnessed the impact of alcoholism and unhealthy relationships among her parents that resurfaced in her own relationship with my dad. This generational curse, as she called it, did not deter her from caring for her three children with an 11th-grade education and as the head of our household. She mastered making something out of nothing. Despite being well dressed and referred to by friends as "Hollywood," she lived a life unfairly marked by struggle. As one of the few family members to ever own a home, she extended a warm welcome to anyone who needed it. She did not live to see me continue her legacy by purchasing my own home. Her diagnosis was cancer, which cut short my grandmother's life, too. What was never documented in either of their medical charts was the weight of racism.

The impact of structural racism on the health of Black women is well-documented (Bailey et al., 2017; Gee and Ford, 2011; Jenkins, 2019; Wallace et al., 2017). We observe how healthcare and educational systems are designed to fail us—from implicit bias projected on Black women in medical offices to adultification bias projected onto Black girls in principals' offices (Epstein, Blake, and Gonzalez, 2017; Morris, 2015). The coronavirus pandemic has laid bare what structural racism looks like in healthcare settings, workplace practices, and living conditions that make Black women (and other historically marginalized populations) more vulnerable to the coronavirus, or the 'Rona as it is colloquially referenced. Throughout this chapter, I use the terms coronavirus, 'Rona, and COVID-19 interchangeably.

During a coronavirus White House briefing on April 10, 2020, the U.S. Surgeon General Jerome Adams addressed the nation urging Black communities to stop using drugs as an effective strategy to curb the disproportionate rates of new coronavirus cases we face. This plea—from a Black man to Black people—to "do it for Big Momma" fell on deaf ears as many critics shunned his since rescinded message. For some, these words may have conjured up the stereotypical images of a Black mammy. In this chapter, I defy these racist and sexist undertones by honoring and applying the title "Big Momma" to the real and perceived ways that Black women engage in other-mothering to protect and advance our health and well-being in the face of racist and patriarchal structures.

In particular, I write about the work of the following Big Mommas: Dr. Joia Adele Crear-Perry (Founder and President, National Birth Equity Collaborative), Dr. Venus E. Evans-Winters (Founder, Planet Venus), and Tricia Hersey (Founder, the Nap Ministry). I ascribe this title and symbolic gesture of respect to these Black women for stepping into the gap left by health and educational systems to provide the healing, stories, and refuge that Black girls and women need to thrive. These Big Mommas engage in other-mothering by creating and sustaining intergenerational legacies for other Black women to relate, relax, resist, and recharge. This is necessary for us to survive the 'Rona.

I recognize the historical, social, and cultural connotations attached to describing Black women as caregivers. This description does not always reflect autonomy and rights. For instance, there is a sordid history of Black women being coerced into caregiving roles that required them to breastfeed white women's babies throughout chattel slavery that has morphed into a unidimensional mammy trope. When I write about mommas, I am pulling on the idea that Black women are at the center of many Black families and communities. We often serve in a caregiving, or other-mothering, capacity whether or not we birth children of our own. I revisit the concept of other-mothering in subsequent sections.

The matriarchal role of other-mothering comes in many forms, from our historical Big Mommas to the more contemporary "aunties". Regardless of the term of endearment used, the role remains the same: to serve as the primary source of psychosocial support for the family and community—which gets taken up in writings on the mundane realities of Black women, or womanism (Davis, 1972). One of our Black women ancestors, bell hooks, captured how we take on social roles as servant-leaders in the *Sisters of the Yam* (1993) as does Cherrie Morago in *The Bridge Called My Back* (2015) in an anthology she co-edited with Gloria Anzaldúa that reminds me of the psychic struggles my mother endured attached to her many thankless roles that was passed down to her from my grandmother. It is the ability of Black women to both survive and thrive that I see, respect, admire, and value as community praxis.

The lived experience of Big Momma fuels her own reflective action, or praxis, that we can continue to carry in our own stories. Community praxis serves as a form of resistance to the racism in our midst. I highlight these three symbolic Big Mommas (and the legacies they extend) to offer lessons on how to disrupt racism and its threat to health equity. It concludes with how leaders can draw on the ancestral knowledge of Big Mommas to fill an important gap in addressing the structural inequities that attempt to limit opportunities for health for Black girls and women—especially during a triple pandemic of racism, state-sanctioned violence, and the 'Rona.

Surviving racism, gender oppression, ableism, and other forms of systemic oppression present a hard, long, painful life for Black women and the communities we love. Yet, we remain the most educated group in the United States leading grassroots and legislative efforts to defy voter suppression, reproductive injustice, police brutality, and educational disparities. We care for our communities in ways that can include our physical bodies but in ways that often extend to our spiritual warfare, our mental fortitude, emotional intelligence, and intellectual faculties. I use an other-mothering lens to describe Big Momma as a philosophy of health that shapes how we think about and narrate research on Black girls' and women's health.

This chapter opens with a description of (a real or symbolic) Big Momma. I write about Big Momma in the singular and plural form depending on its use but the context remains unchanged. This exploration first defines the role Big Momma plays in the family and community, before unpacking how she has had to care for herself and community.

BACKGROUND

It is important to first describe Big Momma—relationally, semantically, culturally, and symbolically. It is the symbolic nature of a Big Momma that allows for me to expand into the concept of other-mothering in this section. I close with the legacy of other-mothering.

The relationship to Big Momma varies. In short, not everyone has one. And, for those who do, the relationship to them can vary from their grandmother, great-grandmother, and/or great-great-grandmother on one or both sides of their families to others who take on grandmotherly roles. But who qualifies as a momma or grandmother is not always limited to the family. This is why some great-aunts could indeed serve and be revered as a Big Momma. Community "mommas" like the women elders who care for other people's kids may also find themselves as honorary grandmothers and called Big Mommas.

From the spelling to the terminology, the concept of a Big Momma (also spelled "mama") is not universally applied in Black families across the Diaspora. If one's family does use this reference, its use not only indicates a sign of respect but the name itself serves as a term of endearment. This explains why some families would refer to their Big Mommas as madear (short for "mother dear" and often pronounced "madea"). The other terms Black families may use to show respect, honor, and love for this maternal figure is through the use of the terms "momma dear," "big ma or muh," and "big mo." And, still others, do not refer to these maternal figures as a Big Momma but as "mom," "mema," "mawmaw or mahmah," "mamoush," "g-ma," "g-mom," "grandmom," "grandma," "gran," "granny," "grandmother," "GG or Gigi," "gramgram," "grammy," "nan," "nana," "nanny," "abuela," and "aunt (insert first name)." Some grandmothers have unique names given to them like "glam-mom" or what my nieces called my mom, "Mimi."

Through informal conversations with Black women, I learned that the use of the term "Big Momma" takes on a cultural tone. There are Black women across the African Diaspora who do not use the term "Big Momma" though they may very well have an equivalent figure in their families. For instance, one Black woman told me that her family referred to their Big Momma as "lil mama" because of her petite stature, which is very telling of the role of physicality in how the term is applied. This is especially pronounced in the critique that Wilson offers on the capitalistic culture of hip hop as he describes Lil' Kim's alter ego in her song, "Big Momma Thang" (Wilson, 2016). Standing at 4'11," Lil' Kim refers to herself as a Big Momma because of the respect it commands. Big Momma is a person, a role, a cultural reference, and a symbolic gesture. Its symbolism resonates most with me.

We can see how the matriarchal figure of Big Momma has resurfaced in new and useful ways. Case in point, my social networks refer to "our forever first lady," Michelle Obama, as an auntie. The auntie title in many ways parallels what Big Momma represents—wisdom, grace, fortitude—and therefore a woman who inspires and molds you. An auntie can be your momma's sister or her best friend but also, as Sotirin and Ellington write, a woman who is a surrogate mother that you have never met but admire (Sotirin and Ellingson, 2013). The Nigerian-born scholar, Njoki Nathani Wane uses autoethnography to reflect on her own mothering practices alongside those of indigenous women. She historicizes mother work as a mutually agreed upon "other-mothering" (Wane, 2000, p. 105). I like the way she writes about other-mothering as rooted in African traditions reflecting collectivist values to care for children other than your own. She goes on to include "community mothering" (p.112), which parallels my own understanding of how Big Momma is most certainly not limited to one's biological family.

BIG MOMMAS' WORK

Now that I clarified how I view Big Mommas as other-mothers for the larger Black community, I turn to three specific Black women who care for me professionally, academically, and personally. I start with how they self-identify before translating how their persistent, courageous, and renewing spirits deserve recognition as Big Mommas who ignite in Black girls and women to care for ourselves.

Thought Leader. Fighter for Justice

As a licensed Ob/Gyn, Dr. Joia Adele Crear-Perry describes herself as a thought leader on racism and fighter for justice. I have attended plenty of her talks and could not agree more. She always opens with a critique of her own medical school training that characterized a patient's Black race as a risk factor to explain poor health outcomes. She maintains that it is this type of race-based medicine that becomes erroneously practiced as evidence-based medicine. The widespread belief that Black bodies do not feel pain is one of many types of dehumanizing ideologies that led to her current line of inquiry as the founder and director of the National Birth Equity Collaborative and advisory committee member of the Black Mamas Matter Alliance for what Black women need to maintain health. Her body of work, to-date, consistently emphasizes racism—as opposed to race—as the root cause of disparate maternal outcomes among Black women (Crear-Perry, 2016, 2018). I rely on her framing (and persistence) for how I teach and design my own undergraduate health equity curriculum and anti-racism training for practitioners in an academic medical center.

I am attuned to how Big Momma Joia's longstanding message finally rang clear as the nation mourned and protested the killings of Breonna Taylor and George Floyd for many who were previously reticent to name racism as the threat it is (Crear-Perry, 2020). The American Medical Association's (AMA) recent declaration that racism is a public health threat is a long-overdue reckoning of its own legacy of race-based medicine (O'Reilly, 2020). It also sets the foundation for the practice (and training) of evidence-based medicine to be more anti-racist than ever before. While not singularly responsible, I credit the well-established work of Big Momma Joia for contributing to this paradigm shift (Crear-Perry, 2020). She complements and extends the work of other Black women scholars and community health workers, or Big Mommas, such as Camara Jones (Jones, 2000), Dorothy Roberts (Roberts, 1998), Diane Rowley (Hasson et al., 2014), Shawneequa Callier (Bentley, Callier, and Rotimi, 2017), Jameta Barlow (2018), Ndidi Amutah-Onukagha (Mendez et al., 2016), Dara Mendez (Mendez, Hogan, and Culhane, 2014),

Yolanda Lewis-Ragland (Lewis-Ragland, 2021), and Dázon Dixon Diallo (Diallo et al., 2010). Big Momma Joia has not waited for the AMA or other leading medical authorities to get on board. Rather, she charged ahead, leading trainings and coalitions on the impact of racism on health when it was still a contested belief among the medical community.

Truth Teller. Cultural Worker.

If you asked Dr. Venus E. Evans-Winters, who goes by Dr. V, to introduce herself she would tell you that she is a truth teller and cultural worker despite a bio that lists her as a tenured professor of education, a certified psychotherapist, and a licensed social worker. Dr. V (2018) aptly shares how she "writes what I like" as a way to push back against knowledge apartheid. She leads bootcamps to encourage Black girls and women to write about social justice as one of many services she offers to activist scholars through what she calls *Planet Venus* (Venus, 2019). As a youth worker who advocates for voice equity, I gravitate to her message of questioning who gets to determine, contribute to, and access knowledge(s).

My research decisions and burgeoning researcher identity are shaped by emulating the emancipatory practice of Black scholars like Big Momma V. In the same way that she expands what counts as research with field notes filled with poetry and text messages from Black girls, my arts-based participatory action research dissertation study with DC youth relied on cultural artifacts (i.e., photos, hip hop music, bicycles) and visual narratives (i.e., identity maps, data poems) to explore self-identity as urban youth and peer educators (Ward, 2017). The inquiry compares what youth have to say about their own urban youth and peer educator identities with what is said about their identities in public discourses and available literature. The inquiry is based on the belief that a deeper understanding of how youth negotiate their identities as urban youth and as peer educators comes from centering their stories in research. In considering power imbalances and research ethics, the youth received credit for their work at a public art research exhibit they curated and named, "For Us, By Us." As programs and policies normalize the complexities of youth identity as assets within the process of youth development, service providers might meet these youth closer to where they are. As I co-create knowledge with youth in my community-based pipeline program, it is just as important that Black women share and publish our stories so we can learn from, and cite, each other.

Of all of Big Momma V's (2017) publications on the agency of Black girls, the one that I often consider for addressing the tensions of marrying my activist self with my scholarly self is her auto-ethnographic writing on being raised in the image of her Black Panther grandmother. Her upbringing instilled a set of values and awakened a curiosity that grew to affirm her identity in the most disavowing of spaces. Given her story, it was not surprising that she was one of the few scholars nodding along to my presentation at the Hip Hop Literacies Conference where I shared an unpopular critique of the #BlackGirlMagic moniker for inadvertently centering whiteness through the celebration of Black girls and women who defy odds and/or attain white validation (Ward, 2016). Her own writing (2019)—on Black girls not wanting to be heroes, but to be *human*—reflects the trauma-informed lens she brings to her scholarship on the resiliency of Black girls amidst the state-sanctioned violence that pushes them out of school and attempts to confine them to disinvested neighborhoods that we know remain culturally rich. Dr. V complements and extends the work of other Black women scholars and community advocates such as Gloria Ladson-Billings, Beverly Guy-Sheftall, Tamika Mallory, Monique Morris, Valerie Kinloch, and Mindy Fullilove. She, like the other Big Mommas named here, answers her rhetorical question: "Who is taking care of us while we spend most of our time on coaching, uplifting, empowering, [and] taking care of others"? (Evans-Winters, 2019) I respond with the words of June Jordan, "We are the ones we have been waiting for" (Jordan, 2005).

Theater Maker. Community Healer.

The 'Rona has interrupted our collective sense of normalcy. In this time, Tricia Hersey rose to online prominence as the founder of the Nap Ministry, a social media campaign that advocates for rest (Bishop, 2020). I can personally attest to the necessity of her ministry and, therefore, deserving title as the self-proclaimed Nap Bishop. Her social media posts resist the capitalistic social pressure, or grind culture, to treat our bodies as objects, machines, and commodities. Big Momma Tricia admonishes Black girls and women to treat rest as a right to which we are deserving as well as an ongoing act of resistance against dominant cultural norms that suggest otherwise.

While you can call 1-833-LUV-NAPS for a recorded rest message that Big Momma Tricia refers to as "care vibes," what I most appreciate is the re-framing of widespread messages that Black women may internalize on why we need care. She writes, "I'm neither burned out nor an imposter. I live in a white supremacist, capitalist, sexist place that has been reigning terror on me and my entire culture since we landed here via ships. Those are my issues" (Bishop, 2020). Her Big Momma wisdom allows for us to un-learn and re-learn the insidious nature of racialized trauma that calls for us to rest and heal (Hersey, 2022).

Big Mommas care. This care extends to their families, communities, and themselves. This explains why I was especially attuned to the needs of students as they studied-while-Black during emergency remote instruction in a pandemic. Just as Big Momma Tricia creates and shares art as a poet and social activist-based performance artist, I used arts-based education in virtual meetings with my youth peer educators in my youth development pipeline program called Promising Futures (Ward, 2015). She complements and extends the work of other Black women scholars and artists such as Tricia Rose (1994), bell hooks (2014), Valin Jordan (2015), Patricia Hill Collins (Collins et al., 2021), and LeConté Dill (2014). Big Momma Tricia (and the Big Mommas that pour into her) shows us how to use our words, our bodies, and our art as tools and vessels to grow, learn, and resist.

THE COMMUNITY PRAXIS OF SAVING OURSELVES

In a 2018 journal volume, *Speaking for Ourselves: Reclaiming, Redesigning, and Reimagining Research on Black Women's Health*, edited by Black women scholars for Black women scholars, I read about the firsthand account of stress experienced by Cheryl Woods Giscombé as she conceptualized the tenets of the now widely used Superwoman Schema. It was her embodied knowledge that allowed for her to consider the values and beliefs often scripted for, and internalized by, varied Black women. Her schemata offers insights into the impact of chronic stress on Black women who experience both gender oppression and racism as they project strength, suppress emotion, resist dependence, succeed on very little resources, and choose others over themselves. This schema is traditionally used to explain why Black women burn out. While the Superwoman Schema is rooted in intersectional Black feminist thought it has been ironically used to reinforce racist ideas that Black women are superhuman and to blame for caring for everyone's health but our own (Jordan-Zachery, 2017). While some progress is being made, many Black women still internalize unfair and dehumanizing messages that we are indeed superhuman and responsible for the toll of racism in our lives.

A collective other-mothering spurred the re-interpretation of the original Superwoman Schema (Woods-Giscombé, 2010). Similar to how I look to the health and racial equity work of Big Mommas Joia, V, and Tricia, Woods-Giscombé (2018) writes of the influence of her own research mentors (who she describes as foremothers). I can only speculate that their wisdom influenced her to revisit how the Superwoman Schema was not being applied in the ways it was intended—to explain the impact of racism on Black women's health. She has since joined other scholars for an observational cross-sectional study of 206 Black women to uncover how two of the Superwoman domains double as protective factors (Allen et al., 2019). These findings help to understand how Black girls and women survive and/or thrive despite racism that unevenly structures opportunities for our health.

As I think about and experience what Winters (2020) refers to as "intergenerational fatigue" (p.57), I cannot help but consider why our Big Mommas gritted their teeth, held their breath, and made the sacrifices they did. It was so that we could dig deep to combat—and, in some cases, endure—the incessant environmental racism that attempts to limit our opportunities for health. We make choices based on the resources we have. Many of us live in neighborhoods plagued by lead exposure, food apartheid, low-resourced schools, over-policing, and disinvestment (Bailey et al., 2017). Or, if these social determinants of health are not adversely impacting us, it is the Black tax in the corporate office and/or expected guilt for choosing career over family. It is this blurring of economic and educational lines that has perplexed legislators and elected officials as they read the rising numbers of maternal deaths among Black women. Big Momma Joia reminds us that racism is the experience that all U.S. Black women share (Elo, Vang, and Culhaune, 2014; Rosenberg, Desai, and Kan, 2002).

Regardless of where or how we experience racism, it is exacerbated by gender oppression as well as discrimination attached to our other social identities. The toxicity of this unrelenting stress not only alters our capacity to subsist but can be passed on to future generations. It is here that Big Momma V's work is most applicable. In *Celebrating Twenty Years of Black Girlhood: The Lauryn Hill Reader* (Waters et al., 2018), she notes that our ability to be resilient is merely a survival tool. Whether it is education or health, we are starting to dismiss the idea that we should scrape by or work twice as hard. This behavior ages and kills us unnecessarily, even while the racist ideology that is at its core remains intact.

In an article fittingly titled, "What We Can We Learn from Big Mama?" two Black women reflect on what it means to be Black teachers to Black students when whiteness remains the expected norm (Hayes, Juarez, and Cross, 2012). Veteran teacher—Olivia Smith, or big mama—shares with her granddaughter and newer teacher, Christie Hayes, how her social justice teaching praxis has allowed her to model for students how to resist the messages that suggest that they should assume the ideals of white students to be successful. Christie latched on to big mama's counter story to inform her own teaching. Similarly, Big Momma Tricia creates and shares counter-narratives to underscore healing messages for other Black girls and women to accept the truth about how racism operates, commit to unlearning anti-Black messages that blame and cripple us, and protect our peace in the process.

We can no longer wait for health providers to believe us, medical research to include us, or legislators to protect us, and this is ever more urgent in the era of COVID-19. Big Momma Joia warns that many of the statistics on

Black maternal deaths are grossly underreported because standardized mortality data is not collected (Kotlar, 2019). The *Harvard Law & Policy Review* published this gap with *Black Maternal Health Research Re-Envisioned: With, For, and By Black Mamas* authored by Black women scholars and the research writing group of the Black Mamas Matter Alliance (Aina et al., 2020). This work complements the commentary entitled, *Listen to Black Women* for the type of policy analysis needed that is based on the lived experiences of Black women (Barlow and Johnson, 2020).

Black women have analyzed and proposed policy that speaks to our experiences. One example is the *Black Maternal Health Momnibus Act of 2020*—a comprehensive set of bills put forth by Congresswoman Lauren Underwood, Congresswoman Alma Adams, Senator Kamala Harris, and the Black Maternal Health Caucus. This legislation addresses the social and structural determinants of health by offering a plan to track and monitor racism as the true cause of many poor health outcomes—more specifically, preventable Black maternal deaths. It also recognizes that the health of Black girls and women does not start or stop at a health provider's office. By highlighting overlooked populations of Black women such as veterans and those completing jail and/or prison sentences, it expands accountability to housing and transportation authorities to remove barriers to prenatal and postnatal care—which includes racial bias and discrimination. Racism explains why we are three to four times more likely to die giving birth (Crear-Perry, 2016). Racism will kill us much faster than the 'Rona.

Whether it is Black doulas fighting obstetric violence or Black food justice organizers fighting for land stewardship, our Superwoman domains of strength and independence have saved us. Below are a few examples:

They don't believe our pain and/or symptoms . . . we created:

- Black Women's Health Imperative (founded by Byllye Y. Avery in 1983)
- Black Mammas Matter Alliance (co-founded by SisterSong Women of Color Reproductive Justice Collective and Center for Reproductive Rights in 2013)
- Therapy for Black Girls (founded by Joy Harden Bradford in 2014)

They ridicule us for not eating "right" or being physically "fit" . . . we created:

- Girl Trek (co-founded by Morgan Dixon and Vanessa Garrison in 2010)
- A Black Girl's Guide to Weight Loss (founded by Erika Nicole Kendall in 2012)
- Women Advancing Nutrition, Dietetics, and Agriculture (WANDA) (Founded by Tambra Raye Stevenson in 2016)

They don't report crimes against us or convict our perpetrators . . . we created:

- Me Too (founded by Tarana Burke in 2006)]
- Black Lives Matter (co-founded by Alicia Garza, Patrisse Cullors and Opal Tometi in 2013)
- #SayHerName (co-founded by Kimberle Crenshaw with the African American Policy Forum and Center for Intersectionality and Social Policy Studies in 2014)

They don't invest in our youth . . . we created:

- Promising Futures (co-founded by Maranda Ward, Jylana Sheats, Shanell McGoy in 2002)
- Uniquely You Summit (founded by Shaleah Lachè Sutton in 2009)
- Dinnertable Documentary (founded by Asha Boston in 2014)

This is an abbreviated list of ways that Black girls and women have carved out spaces, organized networks, rallied resources and support, built infrastructure, owned our narratives, altered norms, and created more and new knowledges to define our right to health and ways to maintain it when healthcare and educational systems have overlooked, ridiculed, silenced, and attempted to spirit-murder us. One could even argue that the outlets that Black girls and women have designed have been in direct response to whiteness and to preserve community. Our collective ancestral and communal knowledge combats intersectional forms of structural racism.

WHAT THEY REALLY NEED TO DO FOR BIG MOMMA

What can the government do to protect all Black girls, Black women, and their families? Elected and public health officials can learn from Big Momma. And, so can all research on Black girls' and women's health. Big Mommas recognize the current failure of healthcare and educational systems to serve and protect us and offer some level-setting values for elected leaders and researchers to first tackle racism before getting a handle on widespread chronic disease and the 'Rona.

More often than not, structural inequities such as poverty, disinvestment, and discrimination are characterized within educational and policy-based public health efforts as issues of personal responsibility. Big Mommas recognize how this neoliberal rhetoric is particularly detrimental to the health of Black girls and women and have debunked theories that maintain us as the problem. To truly advance Black girls' and women's health in equitable, sustainable, and reciprocal ways, we have learned from our Big Mommas the following foundational truths:

- *Black women have full lives:* Black girls and women are historically pathologized within the so-called "race-neutral" research, science, technology, and policy. Despite claims of gold standard objectivity, there remains bias and self-fulfilling prophecies embedded in research questions and designs, reflected within algorithms and worsened by under-resourced programs and non-inclusive practices. And, these biases harm Black girls and women. Critical race theory invites us to use counter-narratives for this very purpose (Bell, 1995). Big Mommas have shown us how to challenge this form of structural racism by not contributing to the same deficit narratives that we refute.
- *Black women can best speak to their humanity:* The health of Black girls and women is often written about and framed with an overwhelming focus on chronic disease risk and prevalence in ways that dismiss or overlook the psychosocial aspects of health that make Black girls and women fully human. What it means for Black girls and women to be well is not up to white men in lab coats or even hipster yogis who consume Eastern medicine to de-stress. While SisterSong created the national Trust Black Women partnership in 2010 on the right to choose, the concept of "trusting Black women" has turned into a mantra on believing accounts of violence and saving local and national elections. I argue that it should also include Black girls and women defining what counts as health and wellness for them. Big Mommas show us how to come against this form of structural racism by not centering the Westernized and Eurocentric perspectives of medicine, science, and public health that narrowly define health using biomedical markers of disease.
- *Black women are complex and diverse:* The ways that data are collected, interpreted, and used often bring injury to Black girls and women. This is yet another form of structural racism. And, while it is important to collect epidemiological data to identify the scope and depth of the coronavirus pandemic for how it unfairly burdens some communities more than others, that messaging becomes increasingly trite and oversimplified for Black girls and women. The public health surveillance data we use to name health disparities are based on gaps between white populations and everyone else. What remains unquestioned is why white populations remain the comparative reference group for every health outcome to determine norms, outliers, and disproportionality. The University of Maryland's Consortium on Race, Gender, and Ethnicity has pushed back against the colonized ways of collecting and reporting data. They have collated a database that allows researchers to look at nuanced data and within-group differences. This is just one way to

address how data is used to subjugate Black women as a risk population. Big Mommas come against this form of structural racism by not standardizing "whiteness" as the norm to which all other bodies of color are weighed.

Black girls and women aspire to a world we have never seen—one without racism—so we cannot bring the same systems into this uncharted terrain. Big Momma Audre Lorde (1984) made it clear that the master's tools will never dismantle the master's house. We need new tools. One of them is intersectional research. Another Big Momma, Kimberlé Crenshaw (1989), coined the term, intersectionality, and has made inroads in legal studies and policy-based work. Researchers and policymakers must do the same because our identities are complex. It does a disservice to our fields and lines of inquiry when we oversimplify the nuances of human behavior or use erroneous proxies for what we do not take the time to adequately and fully assess in all of its messiness.

So, who is Big Momma? One may think that the answer depends on the generation in which you were born. Or, that its use demonstrates that you were raised in the U.S. South. Some may reflect fondly on this term of endearment for what it means to be bestowed such an honorable title. While others may argue that it is actually a concept unused in their families but instead relegated to a stereotypical woman caricatured in movies. Regardless of where one lands with how they have come to understand or apply the term, title, and role of Big Momma, one thing is clear: There is much utility in who Big Momma is, can be, and the role she serves for the Black family and, by extension, the Black community.

We can translate Big Momma's intergenerational knowledge and communal spirit into policy, practice, research, and cultural change. The world stands to benefit from the foundational truths attached to the being and work of Big Momma as other-mothering community praxis. This work is underway, thanks to so many Big Mommas, including Dr. Joia, Dr. V, and Tricia. Now that we elected the first Black woman as the Vice President of the United States, we know no limits to what is possible for the lives and livelihoods of Black girls and women.

NOTE

1. I am Jan's daughter, the daughter of BessieFaye. Both had southern roots. They knew struggle, pain, and sacrifice. Theyalso knew love, pride, and joy. I dedicate this work to them and the wisdom andknowledge they instilled in the Black women and girls in our family that I nowcarry into my philosophy of health. I also want to thank and acknowledge someof my sista scholars who supported me in the writing of this paper. Iappreciate the biweekly check-ins with Dr. MichelleMeggs. She kept

me accountable and motivated during a tumultuous pandemic andhistorical election. I am also grateful to two online communities, the *Black Ladies in Public Health* and *Binders Full of Black Women and BlackNonbinary People in Academia*. Both mediums allowed me to engage in informalconversations on Big Mommas with colleagues across the Diaspora.

REFERENCES

Aina, A., Asiodu, I., Castillo, P., Drayton, C., Aka-James, R., Mahdi, I. K., Mitchell, N., Morgan, I., Robinson, A., Scott, K., Williams, C., Aiyepola, A., Arega, H., Chambers, B., Crear-Perry, J., Delgado, A., Doll, K., Grayson, N., Jackson, A., and Wolfe, T. (2020). Black maternal health research re-envisioned: Best practices for the conduct of research with, for, and by Black mamas. *Harvard Law & Policy Review*, 14, 393–415. https://harvardlpr.com/wp-content/uploads/sites/20/2020/11/BMMA-Research-Working- Group.pdf.

Bailey, Z. D., Krieger, N., Agénor, M., Graves, J., Linos, N., and Bassett, M. T. (2017). Structural racism and health inequities in the USA: Evidence and interventions. *The Lancet*, 389(10077), 1453–63. https://doi.org/10.1016/S0140-6736(17)30569-X.

Barlow, J. N. (2018). Restoring optimal black mental health and reversing intergenerational trauma in an era of Black lives matter. *Biography*, 41(4), 895–908. https://doi.org/10.1353/bio.2018.0084.

Barlow, J. N., and Dill, L. J. (2018). Speaking for ourselves: Reclaiming, redesigning, and reimagining research on Black women's health. *Meridians: Feminism, Race, Transnationalism*, 16(2). https://www.jstor.org/stable/10.2979/meridians.16.issue-2

Barlow, J. N., and Johnson, B. M. (2020). Listen to Black women: Do Black feminist and womanist health policy analyses. *Women's Health Issues*. https://doi.org/10.1016/j.whi.2020.11.001.

Bell, D. A. (1995). Who's afraid of critical race theory? *University of Illinois Law Review*, 4, 893–910. https://sph.umd.edu/sites/default/files/files/Bell_Whos%20Afraid%20of%20CRT_1995UIllLRev893.pdf.

Bentley, A. R., Callier, S., and Rotimi, C. N. (2017). Diversity and inclusion in genomic research: Why the uneven progress? *Journal of Community Genetics*, 8(4), 255–266. https://doi.org/10.1007/s12687-017-0316-6.

Bishop, N. (2020). The Nap Ministry. Instagram photo, October 20.

Collins, P. H., da Silva, E. C. G., Ergun, E., Furseth, I., Bond, K. D., and Martínez-Palacios, J. (2021). Intersectionality as critical social theory: Intersectionality as critical social theory, Patricia Hill Collins, Duke University Press, 2019. *Contemporary Political Theory*, 20(3), 690–725. https://doi.org/10.1057/s41296-021-00490-0.

Crear-Perry, J. A. (2016, September 30). The Black maternal mortality rate in the US is an international crisis. *The Root*. https://www.theroot.com/the-black-maternal-mortality-rate-in-the-us-is-an-inter-1790857011.

Crear-Perry, J. A. (2018, April 11). Race isn't a risk factor in maternal health. Racism is. *Rewire News Group*. https://rewirenewsgroup.com/article/2018/04/11/maternal-health-replace-race-with-racism/.

Crear-Perry, J. A. (2020). Moving towards anti-racist praxis in medicine. *The Lancet*, 396, 451–453. https://doi.org/10.1016/ S0140-6736(20)31543-9.

Crear-Perry, J. A. (2020). (Founder and President, National Birth Equity Collaborative and Board Member, Black Mamas Matter Alliance). Testimony on expecting more: addressing America's maternal and infant crisis, subcommittee on health, employment, labor and pensions and subcommittee on workforce protections, Committee on Education and Labor, U.S. House of Representatives. Text from: Education and Labor Committee. (Date: 01/28/20). Accessed 01/16/21.

Crenshaw, K. (1989). Demarginalizing the intersection of race and sex: A Black feminist critique of antidiscrimination doctrine, feminist theory and antiracist politics. *University of Chicago Legal Forum* 1989, 1, 139–67. https://chicagounbound.uchicago.edu/uclf/vol1989/iss1/8.

Davis, A. (1972). Reflections on the Black woman's role in the community of slaves. *The Massachusetts Review*, 13(1/2), 81–100. http://www.jstor.org/stable/25088201.

Diallo, D. D., Moore, T. W., Ngalame, P. M., White, L. D., Herbst, J. H., and Painter, T. M. (2010). Efficacy of a single-session HIV prevention intervention for Black women: A group randomized controlled trial. *AIDS and Behavior*, 14, 518–529.

Dill, L. J. (2015). Poetic justice: Engaging in participatory narrative analysis to find solace in the "killer corridor". *American Journal of Community Psychology*, 55, 128–135 https://doi.org/10.1007/s10464-014-9694-7.

Elo, I., Zoua Vang, T., and Culhaune, J. F. (2014). Variation in birth outcomes by mother's country of birth among non-Hispanic Black women in the United States. *Maternal and Child Health Journal 18*, 10, 2371–2381. https://www.ncbi.nlm.nih.gov/pmc/articles/PMC4207849/.

Epstein, R., Blake, J. J., and Gonzalez, T. (2017). *Girlhood Interrupted: The Erasure of Black Girls' Childhood.* Washington, DC: Georgetown Center on Poverty and Inequality. https://genderjusticeandopportunity.georgetown.edu/wp-content/uploads/2020/06/girlhood-interrupted.pdf.

Evans-Winters, V. E. (2017). I am my grandmother's child. In *Privilege Through the Looking-Glass.* Leiden, The Netherlands: Brill | Sense. https://brill.com/view/book/edcoll/9789463511407/BP000006.xml.

Evans-Winters, V. E. (2018). W(riting) What I like. https://podcasts.apple.com/us/podcast/writing-what-i-like/id1462811775.

Evans-Winters, V. E. (2019). About. https://www.venusevanswinters.com/.

Gee, G. C., and Ford, C. L. (2011). Structural racism and health inequities: Old issues, new directions. *Du Bois Review: Social Science Research on Race*, 8(1), 115–132. https://doi.org/10.1017/S1742058X11000130.

Hasson, R. E., Rowley, D. L., Blackmore Prince, C., Jones, C. P., and Jenkins, W. C. (2014). The Society for the Analysis of African-American Public Health Issues (SAAPHI). *American Journal of Public Health*, 104(11), 2072–2075. https://doi.org/10.2105/AJPH.2014.104112072.

Hayes, C., Juarez, B., and Cross, P. T. (2012). What can we learn from big mama? *Critical Education*, 3(1), 1–22.

Hersey, T. (2022). *Rest Is Resistance: A Manifesto*. New York: Little, Brown Spark.

hooks, b. (1993). *Sisters of the Yam: Black Women and Self-Recovery*. Routledge.

hooks, b. (2014). *Teaching to Transgress*. New York: Routledge.

Jenkins, W. C., Victor J. Schoenbach, V. J., Rowley, D. L., and Ford, C. L. (2019). Overcoming the impact of racism on the health of communities: What we have learned and what we have not. In C. L. Ford, D. M. Griffith, M. A. Bruce, and K. L. Gilbert (Eds.), *Racism: Science & Tools for the Public Health Professional*. Washington, DC: American Public Health Association. https://doi.org/10.2105/9780875533049ch02.

Jones, C. P. (2000). Levels of racism: A theoretic framework and a gardener's tale. *American Journal of Public Health*, 90(8), 1212–1215. https://doi.org/10.2105/ajph.90.8.1212.

Jordan, J. (2005). *Directed by Desire: The Complete Poems of June Jordan*. Port Townsend, WA: Copper Canyon Press. https://poets.org/poem/poem-south-african-women.

Jordan, V. S. (2015). Confessions of a light-skinned Black girl: An academic misfit. *Urban Education Research and Policy*, 3(1) 52–62.

Jordan-Zachery, J. S. (2017). *Shadow Bodies: Black Women, Ideology, Representation, and Politics*. New Brunswick, NJ: Rutgers University Press.

Kotlar, B. (2019). Maternal Health Task Force (MHTF) Blog. Maternal Health Visionary Spotlight, July 19, 2019. https://www.mhtf.org/category/maternal-health-visionaries-series/.

Lorde, A. (1984). The master's tools will never dismantle the master's house. In *Sister Outsider: Essays and Speeches*. Berkeley: Crossing Press.

Lewis-Ragland, Y. (2021). *Navigating A Triple Pandemic: Healthcare Workers of Color Confront Racism in America, Health Disparities in Medicine & the Trauma of COVID-19*. ISBN Agency.

Mendez, D. D., Hogan, V. K., and Culhane, J. F. (2014). Institutional racism, neighborhood factors, stress, and preterm birth. *Ethnicity & Health*, 19(5), 479–499. https://doi.org/10.1080/13557858.2013.846300.

Mendez, D. D., Thorpe, R. J., Amutah, N., Davis, E. M., Walker, R. E., Chapple-McGruder, T., and Bodnar, L. (2016). Neighborhood racial composition and poverty in association with pre-pregnancy weight and gestational weight gain. *SSM - Population Health*, 2, 692–699. https://doi.org/10.1016/j.ssmph.2016.09.008.

Moraga, C., and Anzaldua, G. (Eds.). (2015). *This Bridge Called My Back: Writing by Radical Women of Color*. Suny Press. Albany, New York.

Morris, M. (2016). *Pushout: The Criminalization of Black Girls in Schools*. New York: The New Press.

O'Reilly, K. O. (2020, November 16). *AMA: Racism is a Threat to Public Health*. American Medical Association.. https://www.ama-assn.org/delivering-care/health-equity/ama-racism-threat-public-health

Roberts, D. (1998). *Killing the Black Body: Race, Reproduction, and the Meaning of Liberty*. New York: Penguin Random House.

Rose, T. (1994). *Black Noise: Rap music and Black Culture in Contemporary America*. Wesleyan.

Rosenberg, K. D., Desai, R. A., and Kan, J. (2002). Why do foreign-born Blacks have lower infant mortality than native-born Blacks? New directions in African-American infant mortality research. *Journal of the National Medical Association*, 94(9), 770–778. https://www.ncbi.nlm.nih.gov/pmc/articles/PMC2594154/

Sotirin, P. J., and Ellingson, L. L. (2013). *Where the Aunts Are: Family, Feminism, and Kinship in Popular Culture*. Waco: Baylor University Press. muse.jhu.edu/book/21708.

Wallace, M., Crear-Perry, J. A., Richardson, L., Tarver, M., and Theall. K. (2017). Separate and unequal: Structural racism and infant mortality in the US. *Health & Place*, 45, 140–144. 10.1016/j.healthplace.2017.03.012.

Wane, N. N. (2000). Reflections on the mutuality of mothering: Women, children, and othermothering. *Journal of the Motherhood Initiative for Research and Community Involvement*, 2(2): 105–116. https://jarm.journals.yorku.ca/index.php/jarm/article/view/2143/1351.

Ward, M. (2016). *#CaptionThis: Conceptualizing the Social Media Discourse for Its School-to-Prison Pipeline Implications on Black girls' Bodies, Power, and Space*. Paper presentation on "'I know I can Learn: Black Girls' Education Matters" panel at the Hip Hop Literacies Conference, Ohio State University, Columbus, Ohio.

Ward, M. (2017). *Youth Constructed Narratives on the Negotiation of Urban Youth and Peer Educator Identities*. The George Washington University, ProQuest Dissertations Publishing. 10263673. https://search.proquest.com/openview/d5607e0118ed698421099d9bb0d43216/1.pdf?pq-origsite=gscholar&cbl=18750&diss=y.

Ward, M. C. (2015). Promising futures: A compelling model of youth work. In B. Kirshner and K. Pozzoboni (Eds.), *The Changing Landscape of Youth Work: Theory and Practice for an Evolving Field* (pp. 167–169). Charlotte: Information Age Publishing.

Ward, M. (2017). *Youth Constructed Narratives on the Negotiation of Urban Youth and Peer Educator Identities*. The George Washington University, ProQuest Dissertations Publishing. 10263673. https://search.proquest.com/openview/d5607e0118ed698421099d9bb0d43216/1.pdf?pq-origsite=gscholar&cbl=18750&diss=y.

Waters, S., Billye, M., Evans-Winters, V., and Bettina Love. B. (Eds.). (2018). *Celebrating Twenty Years of Black Girlhood: Lauryn Hill Reader*. Bern: Peter Lang.

Wilson, S. (2016). Big Momma Thang. In *Great Satan's Rage: American Negativity and Rap/Metal in the Age of Supercapitalism*. Manchester: Manchester University Press. https://www.manchesterhive.com/view/9781784991845/9781784991845.00.

Winters, M. F. (2020). *Black Fatigue: How Racism Erodes the Mind, Body, and Spirit*. New York: Berrett-Koehler Publishers, Inc.

Woods-Giscombé, C. L. (2010). Superwoman schema: African American women's views on stress, strength, and health. *Qualitative Health Research*, 20(5), 668–683. https://doi.org/10.1177/1049732310361892.

Woods-Giscombé, C. L. (2018). Reflections on the development of the superwoman schema conceptual framework: An intersectional approach guided by African American womanist perspectives. *Meridians: Feminism, Race, Transnationalism*, 16(2), 333–342. https://muse.jhu.edu/article/696146.

Chapter 13

Our WISH for Black Girls' and Women's Health

Women, Intersectionality, Science and Health (WISH) Writing Lab

Breya Johnson, Toni Junious, Martha Kakooza, Carlysha Isaac, Juliette Garofolo, Danielle Whyte, Madelyn Stalter

INTRODUCTION: OUR WISH FOR CHANGE

As students, writers, scholars, sisters, and thought starters, we each bring our own desires, hopes, and dreams to our work. We joined the Women, Intersectionality, Science and Health (WISH) lab to be in community with other women who want to write/right women's health and well-being. Through dialogue, collaboration, and accountability, the WISH lab is a space where we create and outline our wishes for empowering Black women's and girls' health and actions needed for our collective wish to be granted. Many of us have only attended predominantly white institutions (PWIs) where spaces to only talk about Black people were few, and spaces to talk about Black women were fewer. Just finding time to spend and think with other Black students was critical to our learning journey. But, having a space to talk solely about Black women's health was transformative. We were able to workshop health-related research projects, think through community needs, and learn new relevant information. Spaces like the WISH lab fill in the gaps that a traditional PWI education cannot provide for you. Most importantly, we needed a space to think that was outside of the traditional western education system. The "training" most departments provide are only skilling you up in white supremacist supporting ways but in the WISH lab we do something different.

WRITING BLACK GIRLS' AND WOMEN'S HEALTH

Why we write is just as, or even more, important than what we write. Our individual backgrounds and lived experiences shape our philosophies and fuel our purpose. By sharing our *why*, we are able to show up as our full and whole selves in this work and find common ground as a collective. The university, especially now at a time when conservatives are banning books and attacking Black, ethnic, gender, and disability studies, does not welcome the work we do with open arms. We needed this space because we could feel the tension in our bodies sitting in these courses that we know cannot help Black communities. We care about the health of Black women and girls so we explore every possibility to help create and sustain healthy communities. We write because we have no other options. We don't want to just hear negative health statistics about Black women and girls, so we write, and explore new ways to intervene.

Breya M. Johnson

I came to the Women, Intersectionality, Science and Health (WISH) lab to think through my writing work with the help of Dr. Jameta Nicole Barlow (Dr. J). The WISH lab serves as a support space for students writing our way through the world. It also serves as Womanism in praxis. We gather biweekly and support each other as women working in systems designed to kill, exploit, and overwork us. We gather to process ways to give our work our best without dying from the stress of it all. We gathered as a group of mostly Black women who endured a predominantly white institution (PWI). The WISH lab has helped me reflect on critical questions that inform and impact the way I do my work. A philosophy centered on collective engagement built on our innate ways of knowing. Sitting with and learning from other Black women was invaluable to my journey and every opportunity to workshop ideas and problems made me a better scholar.

Toni Junious

I want Black women and girls to not only survive but thrive in their body, mind, and spirit. Much of Black girls' and women's health research have taken a deficit perspective and often blame individuals for their health behaviors (Kumanyika, 2018). Everyone is good at telling us what's wrong. They treat Black women's and girls' health like negativity is the only possibility and this deficit approach is killing us. However, through my work I strive to address the systemic and deeply rooted issues, such as gendered racism, that are determinants of Black women's and girls' poor health outcomes. Black women's and girls' wellness is the commitment to care and wholeness toward oneself. I write to center the wholeness of Black girls and women by honoring and embracing the different elements of one's emotional, spiritual, mental, physical, and collective well-being.

Danielle Whyte

I write about Black girls' and women's health to break the cycle; a cycle that asserts that the natural state of Black womanhood is one of survival, suffering, sacrifice. Black women and girls deserve to thrive. No more living in a state of, to re-conceptualize the well-known Fannie Lou Hamer quote, sickness and exhaustion. In this absence of sickness and exhaustion, I wish for Black women and girls to experience an abundance of health and revitalization. To this, it's in the hands of activists and policymakers to turn this demand into a reality. My writing serves as the foundation for the education of those in power to understand how this reality came to be and what can be done to change the status quo. Moreover, my work speaks directly to Black women in learning to better understand themselves, as it relates to the subconscious adoption of stereotypes, and in turn, how to better take care of themselves.

Martha Kakooza

I write because of Chimamanda Adichie's *The Danger of a Single Story*. Black girls and women are not a monolithic group and I write to decenter Blackness as a Western Hemisphere construct to uproot perspectives of White supremacy through a Transatlantic understanding of Black girls' and women's health. By offering this perspective, my hope is to bridge transnational Black solidarity that centers Afro-diasporic and African experiences in girls' and women's health. In a feminist revolution, solidarity among women challenges the "imperialist, white supremacist, captialist patriarchy" (hooks, 1984/2000, p. xiv). As an undergraduate student, my annual trips to Uganda for the winter break caused my identity development process to be in flux. The salience of race, gender, citizenship in the different hegemonic norms in each country caused a shift in how I showed up, never fully showing up in each place. My identity development process was one of remembering and re-connecting with myself, spaces, and communities. I consistently lived in an in-between space that is neither the United States nor Uganda. Each place shifting, re-defining, and re-constituting what it means to be a Black woman and services offered for my health and well-being.

Carlysha Isaac

At the center of my praxis, my motivations stem from the hope to cultivate more sustainable communities that could lead to a stronger and more inclusive society. For me, this means focusing on and addressing the colonial origins of Black girls and women/womyn's mental health. I am most interested in employing a global dialogue, as our community spans across the Diaspora. With the present-day Black Diaspora having an ever-evolving landscape, my interests also extend to what mental health means to people from all walks of life. When I first developed an interest in studying and writing about the wellness of Black women and girls, it came from a place of realizing that my academic training originated from the pedagogy of figures who did not look like me. There is a lack of literature surrounding Black girls' and women's health, revealing how fragile our systems are. In order to effectively address the instability of these systems, their foundations must be assessed.

Juliette Garofolo

I am immensely grateful to have begun my undergraduate experience with a professor like Dr. J. Like many, I came into college with high hopes of becoming a doctor. Up until that point, I considered science to be concrete, evidence-based, and definitive. At the time, my philosophy of science was that science is truth. As a white person, I had never been disenfranchised by science. The faces of the field look like mine. My philosophy of science was shattered by Dr. J. as she challenged me to decolonize my white-washed worldview. Through epistemologies of Black feminists and Womanists I learned that there was so much I did not understand about the world I wished to "heal." I became enthralled by the writings of The Combahee River Collective, Alice Walker, and Toni Morrison, whose skillful diction and powerful syntax educated me on the ways that words could be a tool of resistance. I write about Black girls' and women's health because I believe that to bring forth social transformation in the field of Black girls' and women's health, we require the total involvement of every man, woman, and child (Beale, 2008). I write because I feel it is my responsibility as a student of public health to bring attention to methodological biases in science that continue to impede Black girls and women from achieving health equity (Shiriki, 2018).

Maddie Stalter

I write about Black girls' and women's health to address the unnecessary suffering that women, specifically women of color, face in America's medical systems because they aren't valued as highly as other groups. I write because I was given unearned and unmerited privileges in America even before I was born just because of where I was born and to whom I was born, and these privileges have harmed many people mentally, physically, and emotionally. I write to avoid complacency that many white individuals have promoted throughout America's history.

POSITIONALITY: THE PERSONAL IS POLITICAL

Our identity and intersectionality are key influences for our work. We do not have the privilege to separate the personal from the political. Black women and girls experience a double jeopardy of power imbalances due to our simultaneous manipulation, exploitation, and assault by both racist and sexist systems (Beal, 2008). This intersectionality of our marginalized identities creates a unique struggle and oppression (Combahee River Collective, 1983; Williams & Jackson, 2019). Our collective well-being is influenced by these socio-structural factors and our work prioritizes centering Black women's and girls' voices, identity, and lived experiences.

Juliette

Conversations about racial injustice should not be limited to the boundaries of the Black community. Unpacking the history of colonialism, violence, experimentation, and exploitation of Black bodies is a responsibility of all people, especially white people. It is understood that healing Black girls and women will heal all communities. Although I may not be a member of the Black community, as a woman, a daughter, a sister, a feminist, a student, and an aspiring change-maker, I feel it is my responsibility to bring conversations about Black girls' and women's health to the forefront of every discussion. My whiteness provides me with the privilege to center conversations about Black girls' and women's health. This privilege enables me to deconstruct the oppositional gaze toward Black healing and incorporate Black ways of knowing into conversations about health equity. While I myself do not possess a Black consciousness, I can use my privilege to make space for those who do.

Danielle

I'm uniquely positioned to do this work as I specialize in dialogue-based personal deconstruction efforts and self-care and self-actualization practice development. Self-actualization as I define it is the process of understanding that it is not enough to resist, one must radiate. To this, radiance is the state of radical self-acceptance. An acceptance of self so glowing and bright that it transforms the world around you. Likewise, my wisdom grown from lived experiences have significantly influenced my positionality as a Black woman.

Carlysha

Many of our Black movers and shakers were also global collaborators, and I drew a great deal of inspiration from this. Angela Davis, for example, completed her doctorate degree at the Humboldt University of Berlin, the same school where WEB DuBois completed his master's degree. This is not to say that receiving education abroad is the answer; however, I think there is something to be said about our experiences that can be realized once we step out of the American bubble. Having been racialized in the United States, followed by the opportunity to receive an education abroad, has shaped my philosophy toward wellness and its possibilities. When I was living and studying in Ireland, I was exposed to a different healthcare system. While not perfect, it allowed me to better understand what healthcare and welfare could be like with more accessibility and inclusivity. As a Black woman writer and scholar, I have postured myself to be comfortable with consistently asking, *why?* Why do our institutions, such as universities, operate the way they do? Why do they fail us? What can we build in place of this?

In exploring more of the university sphere, there are a number of contrasts between my experiences in the United States and abroad. While living in Ireland, I learned that one's healthcare was not linked to their student or employment status. This did not apply to me, as I had to pay for my own healthcare insurance as an international student. However, the process in which I sought medical attention was similar to how any citizen would utilize Ireland's universal healthcare system: I was able to go to a clinic, see a doctor, receive treatment within that same day — all with little to no copayment. My experience with healthcare while attending school in the United States, however, was tied to the status of my parents' employment. Unfortunately, this is not an uncommon story and it is one that has amalgamated into my passion for accessibility in health and wellness, especially for Black women and girls.

Martha

The context of higher education provides the backdrop of a U.S. cultural canvas that can portray a magnified picture of identity negotiation experiences and their impacts on Black women's and girl's health. In the field of feminist and gender studies, it is now clearly understood that theorizing women's experiences from these multiple angles of vision generates new questions, issues, and interpretations (e.g., hooks, 1994; Hill-Collins, 2000; Mohanty, 2004). These theories have broadened and complicated the analysis of the historical, political, economic, and cultural forces that shape women's differentiated lives. Among the key trends and transformations that have significantly impacted feminist scholarship are transnational and Black feminism. Both perspectives theorize across national boundaries and emphasize the significance of historical legacies and contemporary political, economic, racial, and cultural processes that intersect and shape women's lives across time and space, including the particular agendas of diverse feminist movements.

Pioneered by women of color located in the Global North looking to locate their positions as immigrants from the Global South, transnational feminism honors the duality of both lived experiences (Hundle et al., 2019). Therefore, transnational feminist theory emphasizes the situations of women in multiple geographic contexts through the decentering of both national and neo-colonial power structures (Mohanty, 2004). In addition, the theory aims to decenter Western ways of knowing and disrupt embedded hegemonies of nationalist ideologies (Hundle et al., 2019). Both Black Feminist and transnational feminist perspectives can be used to critically examine the connections within a hegemonic educational system that has historically valued the perspectives and knowledge of the dominant White, heterosexual, upper-class, male (Robinson & Franklin, 2011). My narrative will use a transnational feminist framework to demonstrate the complexities of Black women and girls health at the intersections of sexism, racism, and nativism found within the informal structures of higher education.

Despite being exposed to Black Thought from the African Diaspora, I could not fully contextualize the lived experiences of living as Black in the United States. In Zora Neale Hurston's essay *How It Feels to Be Colored Me*, she says that her identity as a "colored" person came alive when she was thrown against a sharp, white background. It is that sharp, white background that mandates the tactical assertion of Blackness in the United States. The academy was the white, gendered, and heteropatriarchal space that was my sharp background.

I became very aware of my "difference" with the subtle differences in the way I was treated and spoken to/of in the United States. I was thrown into an "order" that I was forced to become accustomed to. My skin tone began to hold meaning that sculpted my everyday experience not unlike what I experienced growing up in Uganda. The dynamics of power, and the intraracial experiences played out in ways I was not used to and caught me off guard. In the vignettes that follow, I attempt to tease out my experiences of Blackness of being othered in the academy. When I first arrived in the United States, I moved into a residential hall that was comprised mainly of international students. During our first floor meeting, we were asked to fill out a couple of forms presented back to the resident assistant(RA). This was the first time I was filling out a demographic survey that asked for my racial identity. I scanned through the paper, looking for an identity that fit my understanding at that time. Besides Black was a forward slash with African American next to it and below that was "other." I opted for "other" and scribbled next to it, African. Even after a couple of weeks of international student orientation, no one had mentioned race and its social implications in U.S. society. With a hint of pride at being the first to finish, I took the form to the RA. In a slow, condescending tone, she informed me that I was Black, not African, and asked me to refill the form with no explanation. I turned around hoping to find solace in anyone else on the floor that had kinky twists like mine but there was none. It was not that I was unaware that my skin was the color of deep ebony. It was the tone, the resistance, and the othering I felt in that moment that became attached to my Blackness in the United States. In their article, Gatwiri and Anderson (2020) contend that when Black Africans migrate to Western and settler-colonial societies, they become "objects of curiosity" not only for the white gaze but for society in general. As individuals from a wide variety of cultural, ethnic, and national backgrounds, we are often relegated to singular categories such as "Black"—labels by which many never have previously identified with as my vignette offers. Therefore in addition to becoming hyper-visible as a Black body in a predominantly white space, as an African migrant I also experienced a paradoxical opposite; that of becoming invisible due to my non-Western identification. This led me to appropriate notions of "strangerhood" and denial of belonging to my racial identity as Black impacting my wholeness of self. With an increasing number of Black women and girls enrolling into institutions of Higher Education at varied levels, there still needs to be an understanding of how to support BWGH. In my naivety, I thought Historically Black Colleges would provide the space to be whole and Black. Unfortunately, the microaggressions still continue.

Breya and Toni

All of these individuals lived experiences and insights uniquely position us to write about Black women's and girls' health. Our positionality makes us similar yet also different from one another and the Black women and girls we write about. Recognizing our relative positions of power demonstrates how the personal shapes our understandings and writings.

OFFERING OUR GIFTS TO UPLIFT BLACK GIRLS' AND WOMEN'S HEALTH

Each of us brings a unique gift to righting Black women's and girls' health. Whether it is sisterhood or storytelling, our gifts are a tool to reclaim, redefine, and reconnect to radical and holistic pathways to liberation.

THE GIFT OF SISTERHOOD

Danielle

As a Black woman writer and scholar, I can offer Black women and girls kinship, and an example of what it looks like to live in acknowledgment of your radiance. "No man is an island," and creating safe relational communities are the first step to ensuring healthy communities. To further conceptualize this point, using the wisdom of a Black woman, "[W]e need Black girl friends more than other races of women need friends who are the same race...We share a history and experiences different from other women of other races. Our color is more than just similarity, it is a bond (Hughes & Heuman, 2006, p. 37)" (Davis, 2015, p. 27). Black femme scholars are uniquely positioned to "get" the struggle, and, in turn, give the support that only Black women and girls can give other Black women and girls.

THE GIFT OF STORYTELLING

Toni

As a Black woman writer, scholar, and wellness practitioner, I offer the power of storytelling. As a holistic health practitioner, I am able to curate safe spaces for women to show up for themselves and be in sisterhood with one another. By telling their own stories, they are able to reclaim their liberation of body, mind and spirit. It is imperative for Black women to reclaim their health, rewrite their stories, and revolutionize wellness into a holistic, culturally responsive and community-based healing system. Womanist approaches to health research and interventions, such as storytelling, are needed to address the unique gendered and racial oppression Black women and girls experience. Sharing and documenting Black women's and girls' stories allows us to tap into another way of knowing and create culturally responsive programs that center love, care, and compassion as essential pillars to Black women's and girls' holistic health and healing. Black women's wellness should be told from a position of strength to create programs that build upon their assets and enhance their well-being in meaningful ways.

The practice of sisterhood and storytelling are not exclusive to Black women and girls. However, these gifts are part of our innate ways of knowing that bring us a sense of belonging, community, and healing that uniquely impact our collective well-being. There is power in storytelling. Black women and girls (re)telling their own stories disrupts and redefines the gaze for themselves. Through sharing their common lived experiences, Black women are able to pass down essential wisdom, not only for survival but also healing, to each generation forward.

REIMAGINING BLACK GIRLS' AND WOMEN'S HEALTH

We must reimagine how we address Black women's and girls' health. Through centering our voices and needs, releasing stigma, and redefining strength, we can decolonize our physical, mental, emotional, spiritual, and collective health. It is imperative to cultivate equitable, accessible, and sustainable approaches to Black women's and girls' health while integrating Black Feminist and Womanist perspectives that consider our whole selves and collective wellness.

CENTERING BLACK WOMEN AND GIRLS

Juliette

Black women's health is "intimately connected to the health of the whole community" (Nnawulezi &West, 2018). The American healthcare system was founded on principles of racism, colonialism, and inequality that were created to ensure Black women would never experience equal participation in society. We must push for the use of Black feminist therapies because Black feminist perspectives allow Black women to understand how the internalization stereotypes and notions of Black womanhood contribute to negative health outcomes (Jones & Harris, 2019).

Maddie

We can reimagine BGWH by focusing on individual needs, feelings, experiences, and shared concerns of Black women. This can look like asking Black women questions such as: "What do you want and need right now and how can we advocate for it?" There needs to be less of a focus on pathologizing Black women's health and categorizing women's experiences and an increased focus on the holistic experience of being a Black woman in America.

There needs to be a way to promote community-based research to ensure that research is being performed in a way that promotes Black women's autonomy and in a way to improve community health rather than being performed to advance someone's career in academia. If research is being done on Black women's health, then Black women need to be involved in the entire research process rather than having other groups control the research narrative. Since academia has a long history of corruption and mistrust, the community being researched needs to have a voice to help form a stronger foundation for ethical research that is being done to promote the wellness of the community. There needs to be a greater focus on academics' and researchers' motivations behind their career. Every researcher and academic involved in BGWH needs to be asked why they are participating in a research study to make sure that Black women and girls health is at the forefront of everyone's motivations. BGWH needs to be led by Black women and other impacted individuals and not by other groups of people who wish to look informed and progressive.

Another way to reimagine BGWH is to offer a supportive space for Black women to get in touch with and reclaim their femininity and women's innate intimate relationship with nature. Being in touch with nature can help ground women in their innate abilities such as nurturing, loving, healing, and peacemaking. Focusing on Black women's divine femininity can offer a positive and joyful lens for looking at BGWH. It also creates an environment of kinship between not just other women, but with all forms of life. This lens also supports being present rather than doing and promotes ideas of reclaiming rest, embracing sensuality, and self-love.

A 2018 study looking at ways to support women and girls fitness and wellness journeys found that gender roles, stereotypes, and societal narratives heavily focused on women's bodies have impacted the widening gap between women's and men's physical activity levels (Guthold, 2018). Since all of these factors contribute to women's and girls' complex relationships with physical activity, another study tried a new method called photovoice, where participants are asked to take photos to represent their relationship with health and wellness (Spencer, 2018). This method was used to see if there were any similarities in the environment where women and girls exercise, the type of exercise they regularly participated in, and the overall tone that women have toward health and wellness.

After the seven photovoice submissions were in and discussed amongst the participants, they found that many women seek to challenge gender norms of physical activity through engaging in activities that aren't as traditional such as aerial circus skills and climbing trees (Spencer & Kirk, 2018). However, the major similarity between them was their shared importance on having relationships and support with friends and family as well as their value on being outside in nature to promote health and wellness (Spencer & Kirk, 2018). Photovoice submissions contained many photos of the participants and loved ones spending time with elements of nature such as flowers, trees, and water (Spencer & Kirk, 2018). Although this study didn't intend to look at the relationship between women and nature, researchers found that "nature provides an important context for women to feel comfortable, safe, and confident to navigate the complex gender norms around physical activity" (Spencer & Kirk, 2018). Now more than ever, there is a disconnect between humans and nature due to industrialization and urbanization, which is preventing women from reaping the health benefits of having a close relationship with nature, so what can be done to promote this relationship? How can we promote safety for women who want to get closer to nature?

Danielle

There needs to be a reorientation of our approach to the physical, mental, emotional, and spiritual health of Black women and girls. The current medical system operates off of archaic assumptions and the exclusion of the voices of the very patients, Black women, they claim to center. These assumptions are largely based upon the Strong Black Woman archetype, which can be defined as, "the intersectional cultural assumption of strength as an innate feature in Black women." Often Black women and girls report experiencing repeated instances of medical bias and are not seen for who they are as individuals but, instead, as who they are presumed to be as a collective (Okoro et al., 2020). In reimagining the health and wellbeing of Black girls and women, we must reevaluate who is serving our community and address the power dynamics in healthcare that further alienate us.

RELEASING STIGMA

Carlysha

Black girls' and women's health should be viewed as an integral part of our daily lives. We need to move away from considering this as an afterthought, but rather a value that should be automatically integrated into our institutions. With regard to Black mental health and wellness, this can be reimagined in the work of decolonizing mental health and making it more accessible. Black people make up less than 2 percent of members of the American Psychological Association (American Psychological Association, 2017) as well as making up 3 percent of U.S. therapists (Gaines, 2021). This draws a number of concerns. Many Black people who seek mental health services often seek it out from professionals who are also Black (Gaines, 2021). This may result in long waitlists and professionals experiencing burn-out. Additionally, with Black mental health professionals being a disproportionate minority in this field, there needs to be ways to ensure that other non-Black practitioners have enough cultural competency for the health and wellness of their Black clients. Having a narrative across the Black Diaspora is vital, in that it ensures that we are working toward making Black girls' and women's health more available and sustainable on a global level. Ogbevoen also shared that there is still a lot of negative attitudes toward seeking therapy in the Black community, such as being viewed as a sign of weakness in a person (Malekmian, 2020). Through decolonizing mental health, we can reimagine spaces and approaches to mental wellness that release Black girls and women from the colonizing stigma of mental health.

REDEFINING STRENGTH

Toni

We can reimagine Black girls' and women's health by redefining strength. Strength for Black women and girls is defined as having an unmatched resilience and ability to survive (Carter & Rossi, 2019). While strength has the potential to be empowering, it has also been marginalizing. However, strength as a monolith is damaging and leaves little flexibility to express one's boundaries, self-care, or feelings of sadness, depression, and anxiety (Woods-Giscombe & Black, 2010). Through this approach, Black girls and women became conditioned to neglect one's own needs to prioritize the caring of others in the name of strong womanhood (Carter & Rossi, 2019). Black femininity has been tied to caring for others over oneself; however, this ideal has been silently killing our women and girls.

Thus, prioritizing self-care is a revolutionary act for Black women and girls that is necessary for holistic health and wellness. Self-care can be life-saving. Rest, eating healthy foods, and mindfulness are all self-care practices that can help prevent stress on the body and mind, and reduce poor health. An essential Womanist way of knowing is "realizing one's own wellbeing is connected to the wellbeing of others" (Banks-Wallace, 2000). Reclaiming Black girls' and women's ways of knowing serve as a path toward enlightenment and freedom. Radical joy and intentional rest is how Black girls and women find meaning and cope with life's stressors to feel whole again. We can reimagine Black girls' and women's health by integrating Black Feminist and Womanist approaches to health that center the everyday experiences of Black women and girls discovering self-love, self-care, sisterhood, and well-being on their own terms. Recognizing ourselves as our number one priority is how strength can transform into intergenerational healing.

BOUNDLESS POSSIBILITIES FOR BLACK WOMEN'S WELL-BEING

Black women and girls must "remember our past, to protect our future." This proverb of the Sankofa is an important Adinkra symbol throughout the African diaspora. It expresses our collective wish to reflect on the knowledge gained in the past and bring it into the present in order to make positive progress. The historical and contemporary legacy of slavery, medical exploitation, and systemic oppression in the United States and across the world have influenced the intergenerational transmission of inequitable health outcomes among Black women and girls (Prather et al., 2018). For Black women and girls, the wisdom inherited from our ancestors and foremothers who have survived these adverse experiences have provided tools for preservation and pathways forward to liberation and healing as a collective.

An essential pathway for addressing Black women's and girls' health includes creating spaces for Black women and girls to share their lived experiences, ideas, and needs. These spaces allow Black women and girls to feel safe to play, rest, create, explore their identity, and commune together. It is imperative to utilize Black women's and girls' strength of sisterhood, empathy, and empowerment to develop safe spaces to just be, practice radical self-care and self-love, and release negative stereotypes and social-cultural pressures impacting their health.

We believe in a global collaborative effort, where Black girls and women share their knowledge and experiences to cultivate a new way of approaching health that removes institutional barriers and emphasizes a more humanistic approach. This would also entail dismantling discriminatory policies and practices by developing standardized trainings for healthcare providers on interpersonal skills and cultural competency. Additionally, integrating methods from other more collective societies to provide comprehensive, holistic health services that are not tied to our employment, parents, or status as students. But rather, Black girls and women are provided access to healthcare and wellness for simply being.

The most revolutionary action that could be taken would be a total paradigm shift; a total disruption of the paradigms that work to perpetuate the systemic harm done to Black women and girls. The current issues that plague Black women and girls did not manifest overnight. Thus, we must work backward so we can move forward. In addressing the past, we can create a better, healthier future for all Black women and girls.

Our group believes that starting from ourselves, embracing storytelling, moving away from deficit approaches, finding the utility of love. We also find it imperative to embrace practices and philosophies that are outside of the American lens. In this, interpersonal skills and cultural competency would be standard.

These are our wishes.

Wishes for a radical future where simply being alive is enough. Where survival is not so difficult. Where our health and wellness is the most important thing both collectively and individually.

Wishes that seem so simple but in this world are considered radical.

REFERENCES

American Psychological Association. (2017). *Demographic characteristics of APA members by membership characteristics.* Retrieved from https://www.apa.org/workforce/publications/17-member-profiles/table-1.pdf

Banks-Wallace, J. (2000). Womanist ways of knowing: Theoretical considerations for research with African American women. *Advances in Nursing Science*, 22(3), 33–45.

Barlow, J. N. (2018). Restoring optimal black mental health and reversing intergenerational trauma in an era of Black Lives Matter. *Biography*, 41(4), 895–908.

Beal, F. (2008). Double jeopardy: To be Black and female. *Meridians*, 8(2), 166–176. Retrieved January 11, 2021, from http://www.jstor.org/stable/40338758

Carter, L., & Rossi, A. (2019). Embodying strength: The origin, representations, and socialization of the strong Black woman ideal and its effect on Black women's mental health. *Women & Therapy*, 42(3–4), 289–300.

Combahee River Collective. (1983). The Combahee river collective statement. *Home Girls: A Black Feminist Anthology*, 264–274. https://mronline.org/wp-content/uploads/2018/11/Keyword20Coalition_Readings.pdf

Davis, S. (2015). The "strong black woman collective": A developing theoretical framework for understanding collective communication Practices of Black women. *Women's Studies in Communication*, 38(1), 20–35. https://doi.org/10.1080/07491409.2014.953714

Gaines, P. (2021, May 27). *Black people are in a mental health crisis. Their therapists are busier than ever.* NBCNews.com. Retrieved February 26, 2022, from https://www.nbcnews.com/news/nbcblk/black-people-are-mental-health-crisis-therapists-are-busier-ever-rcna1045

Hooks, B. (2000). *Feminist theory: From margin to center.* Cambridge, MA: South End Press.

Jones, L. V., & Harris, M. A. (2019). Developing a black feminist analysis for mental health practice: From theory to praxis. *Women & Therapy*, 42(3–4), 251–264.

Kumanyika, S. (2018). Moving from silos to systems in Black women's health research. *Meridians,* 16(2), 238–252. https://doi.org/10.2979/meridians.16.2.05

Nkiru Nnawulezi, C. M. (2018, March 1). West; institutional strategies to promote the health of Black women survivors of intimate partner violence. *Meridians*, 16(2), 276–285.

Malekmian, S. (2020, November 18). *Those seeking black therapists in Dublin find them hard to come by.* Dublin Inquirer. Retrieved February 26, 2022, from https://dublininquirer.com/2020/11/18/those-seeking-black-therapists-in-dublin-find-them-hard-to-come-by

Okoro, O. N., Hillman, L. A., & Cernasev, A. (2020). "*We get double slammed!*": Healthcare experiences of perceived discrimination among low-income African-American women. *Women's Health (London, England)*, 16, 1745506520953348. https://doi.org/10.1177/1745506520953348

Paradies, Y., Ben, J., Denson, N., Elias, A., Priest, N., Pieterse, A., Gupta, A., Kelaher, M., & Gee, G. (2015). Racism as a determinant of health: A systematic review and meta-analysis. *PloS One*, 10(9), e0138511.

Prather, C., Fuller, T. R., Jeffries IV, W. L., Marshall, K. J., Howell, A. V., Belyue-Umole, A., & King, W. (2018). Racism, African American women, and their sexual and reproductive health: A review of historical and contemporary evidence and implications for health equity. *Health Equity*, 2(1), 249–259.

Shiriki Kumanyika. (2018, March 1). Moving from silos to systems in Black women's health research. *Meridians*, 16(2), 238–252.

Williams, W., & Jackson, L. (2019). Feminist/womanist/intersectional approaches to interventions with Black girls and women. *Women & Therapy*, 42(3–4), 226–230. https://doi.org/10.1080/02703149.2019.1622907

Woods-Giscomb, C. L., & Black, A. R. (2010). Mind-body interventions to reduce risk for health disparities related to stress and strength among African American women: The potential of mindfulness-based stress reduction, loving-kindness, and the NTU therapeutic framework. *Complementary Health Practice Review*, 15(3), 115–131.

Chapter 14

The Afterword

Reimagining Black Health

Melicia C. Whitt-Glover, Olivia Affuso, Tambra Raye Stevenson, Jameta Nicole Barlow, Shiriki K. Kumanyika

Black women face a myriad of health challenges that are often compounded by intersecting factors such as structural racism, gender, adverse socioeconomic circumstances, and various forms of discrimination over the life course (Williams & Mohammed, 2013; Chinn et al., 2021). These factors reflect inequities that contribute to significant disparities in health outcomes. Black women experience higher rates of chronic diseases such as hypertension, diabetes, obesity, and certain types of cancers that directly and indirectly impact overall health and well-being (Peters et al., 2014; DeSantis et al., 2019; National Center for Health Statistics, 2023). Black women are also disproportionately impacted by reproductive health issues, including higher rates of maternal mortality and morbidity, where studies have consistently shown that Black women are at a greater risk of dying due to pregnancy-related complications compared to our white counterparts, regardless of income or educational level (Petersen et al., 2019). The alarming disparities impacting Black women, even those with the "right" sociodemographic factors (e.g., high education, high income), suggest a need to identify and address factors that directly and indirectly influence and impact individual behaviors (e.g., policies, systems, environments, sociocultural norms) to effectively address health disparities.

On April 13, 2021 the Council on Black Health (the Council) released the nation's first Black Health Bill of Rights. This declarative document serves as the Council's framework for guiding advocacy, education, research, policy, and practice efforts to advance a national agenda for achieving optimal health (Huber et al., 2011) in Black communities. The Bill was created with people of African descent in the United States in mind, and the Council members and leadership believe the document is critical when calling attention to policies, systems, and environments that negatively impact Black women's access to healthcare, related determinants of health, and health outcomes. The Black Health Bill of Rights helps to center the principles of the importance of focusing on underlying factors that are the cause of health inequities and is designed to remind individuals, policymakers, decision-makers, funders, researchers, among others, that it is *systems*, rather than individuals, that are broken and in need of repair if we are to achieve optimal health outcomes within Black communities. In this concluding chapter, we outline the seven Articles within the Black Health Bill of Rights and discuss how the Articles can inform an agenda to achieve optimal health for Black people, with a particular emphasis on implications for Black women.

ARTICLE 1: WE HAVE THE RIGHT TO A CULTURE OF HEALTH THAT VALUES OUR WHOLE WELL-BEING AND ALLOWS US TO ACHIEVE OPTIMAL HEALTH

The first article in the Black Health Bill of Rights focuses on establishing a culture of health as an essential component necessary to achieve optimal health. The concept of a "culture of health" is a powerful framework that emphasizes the importance of creating a society that promotes and supports the health and well-being of all people within its population. Coined and widely disseminated by the Robert Wood Johnson Foundation, "culture of health" encompasses a comprehensive vision for achieving health equity for everyone (Chandra et al., 2017). It recognizes that optimal health extends beyond just the absence of illness and encompasses various dimensions of well-being, including physical, cognitive, psychosocial, emotional, spiritual, occupational, financial, social, intellectual, and environmental aspects. This holistic approach to risk reduction and disease prevention helps establish and maintain a sense of balance across these dimensions. By working toward a culture of health, we can strive to create conditions that support the overall well-being of individuals and communities.

Central to the concept of a culture of health is the recognition that health and well-being are not solely individual responsibilities, but collective endeavors. It emphasizes shared values for community and population health, lifting up the importance of partnerships and collaborations across different sectors of society. This means engaging not only healthcare systems and providers but also policymakers, businesses, educators, community organizations, and individuals themselves. A culture of health is closely aligned with the concept of collectivism (Triandis, 2018). Collectivism is a socio-political ideology and cultural value system that emphasizes the importance of collective action, cooperation, and the well-being of the community or group over individual interests. It is fundamentally opposite of individualism, which prioritizes individual rights, autonomy, and self-interest, but in U.S. society is blended with the individualistic American culture. Collectivism tends to prioritize the needs and goals of the group over the desires of individuals in ways that are atypical of the prototypical American ideal. The collective may be defined in various ways, such as a family, tribe, community, nation, or a specific social or cultural group. The concept of collectivism can manifest in different forms, including cultural norms, social structures, and political systems.

For Black women, it is crucial that the concept of a culture of health encompasses specific experiences and needs for women as individuals and as members of a community which provides support and solidarity. Historically, Black women have relied on communal networks for support, whether through extended family, friendship circles, or community organizations (Sekaquaptewa et al., 2007). These networks have provided crucial emotional, social, and practical support in navigating systemic challenges and promoting resilience. In a culture of health, particularly one that values and understands collectivism, health-related systems and services are designed to be better coordinated and delivered with all consumers in mind, ensuring equitable access and quality of care. This approach recognizes that different communities have unique needs and challenges, and aims to address those needs proportionately. It seeks to eliminate disparities in healthcare access and outcomes, creating healthier communities overall.

Well-being, defined as one's perception of being comfortable, healthy, and happy, should be characterized by a broad range of factors that contribute to the overall health and well-being of Black women. This includes addressing the social determinants of health, such as systemic racism, discrimination, socioeconomic inequities, and access to culturally competent care (Bailey et al., 2017). Collectivism can play a significant role in promoting the health and well-being of Black women. By recognizing the collective impact of systemic factors on health disparities, collectivism highlights the need for community-centered approaches to healthcare, public health and prevention, and addressing social determinants of health. It can also encourage community-led initiatives, health education, and the sharing of resources to improve the overall well-being of Black women.

By advocating for and promoting a culture of health that values the whole well-being of Black women, in family and community contexts, we can work toward achieving health equity and creating a society where every person has the opportunity to thrive and enjoy optimal health. Practical examples of a research and practice agenda for Black women that value a culture of health include:

1. Conducting comprehensive studies on the social determinants of health that specifically focus on the unique experiences and challenges Black women face. This research can explore factors such as systemic racism, socioeconomic disparities, access to healthcare, and cultural influences on health behaviors.
2. Addressing healthcare provider biases and promoting cultural competence in healthcare settings to ensure that Black women receive respectful, dignified, and patient-centered care. This can be achieved through training programs, policy changes, and ongoing evaluation of healthcare practices to identify and eliminate disparities in treatment.
3. Prioritizing intersectionality in research and practice by acknowledging and addressing the unique experiences and health needs of Black women who may face multiple forms of discrimination based on racial categorization, gender, socioeconomic status, and other intersecting identities.
4. Integrating community voices and perspectives into research design, implementation, and evaluation processes to ensure that the priorities and concerns of Black women are central to decision-making and resource allocation.
5. Advocating for policies that support health equity and social justice for Black women, such as affordable healthcare access, paid family leave, and other policies that address the social determinants of health.

ARTICLE 2: WE HAVE THE RIGHT TO RECEIVE RESPECTFUL AND DIGNIFIED HEALTHCARE

The right to receive respectful and dignified healthcare is a fundamental principle that should apply to every individual, regardless of racial categorization, gender, or any other personal or group characteristics (Beach et al., 2006). In the context of healthcare, people and their families often find themselves in a subordinate role, where healthcare providers hold power and authority based on professional expertise. However, it is essential for healthcare systems to recognize and uphold the intrinsic value of every patient as a human being, ensuring that their basic rights are honored and that care is delivered in a manner that preserves dignity.

For Black women, the need for respectful and dignified healthcare is crucial because we face a range of disparities and challenges that can negatively impact health outcomes and experiences within the healthcare system. One significant area of concern is the disparity in maternal morbidity and mortality rates (Minehart et al., 2021; National Center for Health Statistics, 2023). Black women are at a higher risk of dying due to pregnancy-related complications compared to white women. This alarming disparity persists even when controlling for factors such as education and socioeconomic status, indicating that additional factors beyond access to care are at play.

The near-death experience of Serena Williams following the birth of her daughter shed a national spotlight on the issues Black women often encounter when seeking healthcare. Ms. Williams, a highly recognized and accomplished professional tennis player, had to advocate persistently for the appropriate testing and intervention after alerting a nurse to symptoms of a blood clot. Her experience highlights the pervasive presence of implicit and explicit biases that impact Black women within the healthcare system, which can result in delayed diagnoses, inadequate treatment, and ultimately, detrimental health outcomes.

Addressing these biases and ensuring respectful and dignified healthcare for Black women is paramount (Crear-Perry et al., 2020). Healthcare providers and institutions must acknowledge the existence of implicit biases and actively work to dismantle them. This includes implementing training programs that raise awareness of biases, promoting cultural sensitivity and competence among healthcare professionals, and establishing protocols that prevent discrimination based on racial categorization or any other personal characteristic.

Furthermore, healthcare systems must prioritize the development of strategies and interventions that specifically target the disparities in maternal morbidity and mortality faced by Black women (Petersen et al., 2019). This requires a comprehensive approach that addresses social determinants of health, improves access to quality prenatal and postpartum care, and supports the overall well-being of Black women throughout the reproductive years.

Ensuring respectful and dignified healthcare for Black women goes beyond addressing maternal health disparities. It encompasses all aspects of healthcare, including prevention, diagnosis, treatment, and ongoing care for various health conditions. By creating a healthcare system that values and respects the experiences and needs of Black women, we can begin to eliminate disparities and provide equitable and effective care for all. Practical examples of a research and practice agenda for Black women that help elevate the right to receive respectful and dignified healthcare include:

1. Conducting research to understand and address the specific barriers and challenges that Black women face in accessing respectful and dignified healthcare. This can involve studying experiences of discrimination,

bias, and mistreatment within healthcare settings, as well as exploring factors that contribute to disparities in healthcare outcomes.

2. Developing and implementing training programs for healthcare providers to promote cultural competency, empathy, and respectful communication when interacting with Black women. This can include education on implicit biases, cultural humility, and the importance of patient-centered care.
3. Establishing guidelines and protocols within healthcare institutions to ensure that respectful and dignified care is a priority for all patients, regardless of racial categorization or ethnicity. This can involve policies that explicitly prohibit discrimination, provide guidelines for respectful communication, and encourage patient advocacy and empowerment.
4. Collaborating with community organizations and leaders to raise awareness about the importance of respectful and dignified healthcare for Black women. This can involve community education programs, workshops, and campaigns that aim to address healthcare disparities, promote health literacy, and encourage self-advocacy.
5. Partnering with policymakers and advocacy groups to advocate for policies that protect and promote the right to receive respectful and dignified healthcare for Black women. This can include advocating for policies that address healthcare inequities, promote diversity and inclusion within healthcare settings, and enforce accountability for instances of discrimination or mistreatment.
6. Engaging in ongoing evaluation and quality improvement efforts within healthcare institutions to monitor and address disparities in the provision of respectful and dignified care. This can involve collecting data on patient experiences, tracking healthcare outcomes, and implementing strategies to improve cultural competence and patient satisfaction.

ARTICLE 3: WE HAVE THE RIGHT TO ENGAGE WITH A HEALTHCARE INDUSTRY AND RECEIVE HEALTH CARE THAT IS CULTURALLY SENSITIVE AND THAT INCORPORATES CULTURAL HUMILITY AND STRUCTURAL EQUITY

The right to engage with the healthcare industry and receive culturally sensitive care is essential for Black people. Culturally sensitive health care, also known as culturally appropriate or culturally competent care, recognizes the significance of understanding and responding appropriately to the attitudes, feelings, and circumstances of individuals who share a common and distinctive racial, national, religious, linguistic, or cultural heritage (Betancourt et al., 2003). It involves tailoring healthcare services to meet the specific cultural needs and preferences of patients, ensuring that values, beliefs, and traditions are respected and incorporated into care.

Cultural humility takes the concept of cultural sensitivity further by emphasizing a process of self-reflection and discovery for healthcare providers (Foronda et al., 2016). It calls for providers to continuously examine their own biases, assumptions, and limitations, while actively seeking to build honest and trustworthy relationships with patients. By acknowledging the power dynamics inherent in the patient-provider relationship and adopting a stance of humility, healthcare providers can work to address disparities in care and foster a more equitable healthcare environment.

Structural equity is a critical aspect of ensuring culturally sensitive and equitable healthcare (Bailey et al., 2017). It requires a comprehensive examination and dismantling of systemic barriers that impede equity within the healthcare system (Fiscella & Sanders, 2016). While legal segregation in healthcare has officially ended, significant efforts are still needed to elevate standards to fair and just levels for all people, including Black Americans. This includes addressing issues such as health insurance systems, training of healthcare professionals, and the physical locations where care is delivered. It is imperative to recognize and remove barriers that limit access to and quality of healthcare services for Black individuals.

Achieving cultural sensitivity, cultural humility, and structural equity in healthcare also extends to how Black healthcare providers, researchers, and trainees are treated in relevant settings (Dyrbye et al., 2006). The demands for dignity and respect apply not only to patients but also to those who contribute to the healthcare industry. This involves creating inclusive and supportive environments that value the contributions and perspectives of Black healthcare professionals, ensuring fair treatment and equal opportunities for advancement and professional growth.

To fulfill the right to engage with the healthcare industry and receive culturally sensitive care, it is crucial to implement and enforce stronger and more inclusive policies. This includes actively promoting cultural competency training for healthcare providers, diversifying the healthcare workforce, and developing strategies that address the social determinants of health and systemic inequities. By actively striving for cultural sensitivity, cultural humility, and structural equity, the healthcare industry can create a more inclusive and equitable environment that meets the needs of all people, regardless of cultural background.

Practical examples of a research and practice agenda for Black women that support the right to engage with a healthcare industry and receive culturally sensitive care that incorporates cultural humility and structural equity include:

1. Researching the healthcare experiences and needs of Black women to identify gaps and disparities in culturally sensitive care. This can involve studying the impact of cultural beliefs, practices, and social determinants of health on healthcare outcomes and access.
2. Developing and implementing cultural competency training programs for healthcare providers and staff that focus specifically on understanding the unique cultural backgrounds, histories, and experiences of Black women. This can include education on cultural humility, anti-racism, and addressing implicit biases.
3. Establishing guidelines and protocols within healthcare institutions that promote cultural sensitivity and humility in all aspects of care, including communication, decision-making, and treatment. This can involve incorporating cultural assessments, patient-centered care plans, and ensuring diversity and representation in healthcare leadership positions.
4. Collaborating with community organizations and leaders to co-create culturally sensitive healthcare initiatives and programs that address the specific needs of Black women. This can involve community engagement and participatory research, and also involve community members in the design and evaluation of healthcare interventions.
5. Advocating for policy changes that promote structural equity within the healthcare system. This can include initiatives to address healthcare disparities, promote health equity, and ensure equitable distribution of resources and services in underserved communities.
6. Supporting the development and expansion of community health worker programs and culturally specific healthcare services that prioritize the needs of Black women. This can involve training and employing community health workers who are trusted community members and can serve as liaisons between healthcare providers and Black women.
7. Incorporating cultural humility and sensitivity into healthcare quality improvement efforts, such as patient satisfaction surveys and feedback mechanisms. This can involve actively seeking feedback from Black women and using lived experiences and knowledge as input to drive changes in healthcare delivery and practices.
8. Conducting research on the effectiveness of culturally sensitive interventions and strategies in improving healthcare outcomes for Black women. This can involve evaluating the impact of culturally tailored interventions, community health worker programs, and other initiatives aimed at reducing disparities and improving patient experiences.

ARTICLE 4: WE HAVE THE RIGHT TO APPROACH SOLUTIONS TO BLACK HEALTH FROM A STRENGTHS-BASED APPROACH THAT INCORPORATES A DECOLONIZED AND INTERSECTIONAL LENS TO HEALTH EQUITY

The concept of decolonization is rooted in the history of colonization, where certain populations, such as indigenous communities and Black people, were subjected to control, exploitation, and the denial of our human and cultural rights by external powers seeking to expand their influence and wealth (Czyzewski, 2011; Sium et al., 2012). In the context of race and ethnicity, colonization refers to the subjugation and oppression of indigenous populations and the historical exploitation of Black people in Africa and America by European colonizers.

To address Black health disparities, it is crucial to adopt a decolonized approach that challenges the long-lasting effects of colonization (Adebisi, 2023). This approach recognizes that the impacts of slavery and historical injustices have persisted even after emancipation, shaping the differential experiences and challenges faced by different gender and age groups within Black communities. By acknowledging the intersectionality of these effects, we understand that the health of Black people cannot be viewed as a singular racial issue but as a complex interplay of race, gender, age, and other intersecting factors.

A decolonized approach to Black health equity involves countering biased assumptions, stereotypes, and misperceptions that devalue Black lives and health. It also entails dismantling both overt and hidden structures that limit access to quality education, wealth, and other essential resources necessary for achieving health equity. By challenging and transforming these oppressive systems, we can create a more equitable society where the health and well-being of Black people are valued and prioritized. This book represents ways in which we can engage ontologies and epistemologies to engage more appropriate decolonizing methodologies for Black health.

Moreover, a strengths-based approach recognizes and builds upon the resilience, knowledge, and assets within Black communities. It shifts the focus from solely addressing deficits and challenges to also highlighting the strengths, resources, and cultural heritage that contribute to the well-being of Black people. By centering the strengths and agency of Black communities, solutions can be developed in collaboration with the community by leveraging expertise and lived experiences to promote health equity.

Incorporating an intersectional lens is vital to understanding the multifaceted nature of Black health disparities (Crenshaw, 1989). It recognizes that individuals experience intersecting forms of discrimination and marginalization based on race, gender, socioeconomic status, and other social identities. By adopting an intersectional approach, we acknowledge that solutions to Black health disparities must address the unique challenges faced by different subgroups within the Black community and work toward comprehensive, inclusive, and culturally sensitive interventions. Black women, in particular, face unique challenges that result from the intersection of race, gender, and other factors, underscoring the need for tailored approaches that consider all factors when developing interventions to effectively address health and related factors in Black women.

Practical examples of a research and practice agenda for Black women that support the right to approach solutions to Black health from a strengths-based approach incorporating a decolonized and intersectional lens to health equity include:

1. Conducting research to understand and build on the strengths and resilience of Black women in the face of health disparities and inequities. This can involve exploring the protective factors, coping mechanisms, and community assets that contribute to health and well-being.
2. Developing and implementing interventions that build upon the strengths and cultural assets of Black women and Black communities. This can involve promoting community-led initiatives, culturally relevant health promotion programs, and interventions that leverage existing community resources and networks.
3. Incorporating an intersectional lens in research and practice to understand the unique experiences and needs of Black women based on the intersections of racial identity or categorization, gender, socioeconomic status, sexuality, and other social identities. This can involve studying how multiple forms of oppression and discrimination intersect and impact Black women's health outcomes.
4. Engaging in participatory research approaches that involve Black women as active partners in the research process. This can include community-based participatory research (CBPR) models that prioritize the involvement of Black women in all stages of research, from design to dissemination.
5. Collaborating with Black women-led organizations and community stakeholders to co-create and implement health interventions and programs that are grounded in lived experiences and address population-specific needs and challenges.
6. Challenging and decolonizing traditional research methodologies and frameworks that perpetuate power imbalances and reinforce stereotypes and biases. This can involve adopting research methods that center Black women's voices, knowledge systems, and ways of knowing, such as storytelling, oral histories, and other culturally relevant approaches.

7. Advocating for policy changes that address structural inequities and promote a decolonized and intersectional approach to health equity. This can include advocating for policies that address social determinants of health, promote racial and gender equity, and center the experiences and needs of Black women.
8. Promoting cultural humility and competency among healthcare providers and professionals working with Black women. This can involve training programs that challenge stereotypes, address implicit biases, and foster respectful and empowering relationships between healthcare providers and Black women.

ARTICLE 5: WE HAVE THE RIGHT TO TRANSFORM OUR HEALTH BY RECLAIMING OUR POWER AND AUTONOMY

Building upon the principles outlined in Article 4, Article 5 emphasizes the need for Black people to have the agency, resources, and autonomy necessary to transform health and well-being. It recognizes that addressing health threats and disparities stemming from historical injustices is insufficient. Black communities should have the power to actively shape our own health outcomes and create opportunities for optimal health and well-being.

Central to this Article is the concept of self-determination (Ryan & Deci, 2000), which asserts that Black people have the right to make decisions and control our own destinies regarding our health. This includes having access to the necessary resources, services, and opportunities that enable achievement of the highest health potential. The definition of optimal health should not be limited to a comparison with the health of the white population in the United States, as that standard does not necessarily reflect true optimal health. Instead, optimal health should be determined by the aspirations and needs of the Black community, considering our unique experiences and perspectives (Huber et al., 2011).

Reclaiming power and autonomy in health means challenging the structures and systems that perpetuate health disparities and limit opportunities for Black people to thrive. It involves advocating for equitable distribution of resources, including access to quality healthcare, education, employment, housing, and other social determinants of health. By dismantling barriers and addressing systemic inequities, Black people can assert our agency and actively participate in decisions that impact our health.

Furthermore, Article 5 acknowledges that health is not solely determined by individual behaviors or choices but is deeply influenced by social, economic, and environmental factors. It calls for a comprehensive approach that recognizes and addresses the inequities that are the root causes of health disparities, such as poverty, discrimination, and unequal access to resources. Black communities, including Black women within communities, should be empowered to design and implement interventions that reflect cultural values, knowledge, and strengths, fostering a sense of ownership and relevance.

Practical examples of a research and practice agenda for Black women that support the right to transform health by reclaiming our power and autonomy include:

1. Conducting research on the historical and systemic factors that have impacted Black women's access to power and autonomy in healthcare. This can involve examining how structural racism, sexism, and other forms of discrimination have influenced healthcare practices and policies, and exploring strategies to dismantle these barriers.
2. Promoting community-led initiatives that prioritize the voices and leadership of Black women. This can include supporting grassroots organizations and initiatives that empower Black women to address health issues specific to Black communities, advocate for policy changes, and drive positive change from within.
3. Collaborating with Black women's organizations and community stakeholders to co-design and implement programs that promote self-care, self-determination, and holistic well-being. This can involve offering culturally tailored services, workshops, and support groups that address the unique needs and experiences of Black women.
4. Engaging in research that explores alternative healing practices and traditional knowledge systems within Black communities. This can involve studying the effectiveness of culturally specific healing modalities and integrating them into mainstream healthcare practices, respecting and validating diverse approaches to wellness.
5. Advocating for policies that prioritize the autonomy and agency of Black women in healthcare decision-making. This can involve advocating for informed consent, patient-centered care models, and policies that address the power dynamics and systemic biases that can hinder Black women's ability to make autonomous choices about our health.
6. Promoting representation and diversity in healthcare leadership and decision-making positions. This can involve advocating for increased representation of Black women in healthcare administration, research, policy-making, and other influential roles to ensure that our perspectives and needs are considered.
7. Providing resources and support for entrepreneurship and economic empowerment among Black women in the health and wellness sector. This can involve creating funding opportunities, mentorship programs,

and business development support to foster the growth of Black-owned healthcare businesses and initiatives.

ARTICLE 6: WE HAVE THE RIGHT TO HONOR AND INCORPORATE LESSONS FROM OUR PAST, PRESENT, AND FUTURE AS A PATHWAY TO RESTORING OUR HEALTH

Article 6 of the Black Health Bill of Rights recognizes the importance of acknowledging and learning from the rich history of Black Americans as a means to restore and improve health. It acknowledges the historic resilience demonstrated by Black people and communities in the face of immense challenges throughout history (Utsey et al., 2008). This resilience should be celebrated and recognized, *but it should not serve as an excuse for perpetuating existing health disparities and challenges.*

Central to this Article is the recognition that historical narratives have a profound influence on health practices within Black communities (Paradies, 2006). It emphasizes the need for Black children to learn about the impact of historical events and experiences on present-day health outcomes. By understanding the connections between history and health, future generations can be empowered to address and overcome the lingering effects of historical injustices.

The Article also highlights the importance of recognizing the contributions of Black heroes in health research and healthcare, both in the past and the present (Gamble, 1997). By educating and inspiring future generations about these trailblazers, Black children can see themselves reflected in the health field and be motivated to pursue careers in healthcare and research. This ongoing process of learning and celebrating accomplishments ensures that future achievements are recorded and celebrated, fostering a sense of pride and empowerment.

Furthermore, Article 6 recognizes that there are positive aspects of African and Black American history that can be integrated into current practice (Airhihenbuwa et al., 2014). This includes social and cultural assets, traditions, and lessons that hold value for the restoration of health. By respectfully and safely incorporating these aspects into healthcare and health practices, a deeper understanding of the shared history of African peoples globally can be fostered. This recognition and connection to Black identity, including the African Diaspora, can strengthen bonds and promote a sense of solidarity among Black individuals and communities.

Practical examples of a research and practice agenda for Black women that support the right to honor and incorporate lessons from our past, present, and future as a pathway to restoring our health include:

1. Conducting research that delves into the historical experiences, health practices, and cultural traditions of Black women. This research can shed light on the resilience, knowledge, and wisdom embedded in Black women's history and inform current healthcare practices.
2. Facilitating intergenerational dialogues and knowledge sharing between older and younger generations of Black women. This can be achieved through community-based initiatives, oral history projects, and mentorship programs that aim to preserve and transmit valuable health-related lessons from the past to present and future generations.
3. Supporting research and practice that celebrates and revitalizes cultural practices and traditions within Black communities. This may involve initiatives to preserve traditional healing methods, incorporate culturally relevant dietary practices, or revive and adapt cultural ceremonies that promote holistic well-being.
4. Engaging Black women and Black communities as active participants in the research process. This can involve participatory research methods prioritizing community input, collaboration, and shared decision-making. Community-led initiatives and programs can be developed based on the insights gained from these partnerships, ensuring that research and practice are grounded in the needs, strengths, and aspirations of Black women.
5. Integrating traditional and conventional medicine: Exploring ways to integrate traditional healing practices and knowledge systems with conventional medicine. Research can focus on understanding the effectiveness, safety, and cultural appropriateness of traditional healing practices and developing frameworks for their incorporation into mainstream healthcare systems. This integration can enhance access to culturally appropriate care and improve health outcomes for Black women.
6. Strengths-based interventions: Developing interventions and programs that build on the strengths and resilience of Black women. These may include empowerment initiatives, mentorship programs, and skills-building workshops that promote self-care, self-advocacy, and overall well-being. Emphasizing a strengths-based approach acknowledges the assets and capabilities of Black women and leverages the strengths to improve health outcomes.
7. Policy advocacy and reform: Engaging in advocacy efforts to address systemic inequities and promote policies that honor and incorporate the lessons from the past, present, and future of Black women's health. This can involve advocating for increased funding for research and initiatives that prioritize the health needs of Black women, as well as policy reforms that address social determinants of health and systemic barriers to healthcare access.

ARTICLE 7: WE HAVE THE RIGHT TO HAVE OUR FULL HUMANITY HONORED AND VALUED

Article 7 of the Black Health Bill of Rights emphasizes the fundamental principle that all people, regardless of racial categorization or ethnicity, have the right to have their full humanity honored and valued. It acknowledges that while the principle of equality and human rights should apply universally, the recognition and establishment of these rights for Black people have not been fully realized.

The Article highlights the historical struggle for equal rights and recognition of the full humanity of Black people (Davis, 2005). It acknowledges that constitutional amendments were necessary to grant rights as citizens to Black people, indicating that recognizing our humanity has required specific legal interventions. Despite these advancements, the health statistics of Black communities reflect a failure of American leaders, institutions, and society to fully acknowledge and honor the humanity of Black people (Williams & Mohammed, 2013).

The Article draws attention to the fact that health is a human right and should be treated as such. It acknowledges that there are ongoing challenges related to voting rights for Black people, with implicit and explicit questioning of these rights still present in society. By raising these human rights issues in the dialogue about Black health, the Article aims to shed light on the systemic inequities and biases that continue to affect the well-being of Black communities.

In essence, Article 7 calls for the recognition and affirmation of the full humanity of Black people. It underscores the importance of addressing the historical and current injustices that undermine the realization of this fundamental principle. By advocating for the equal value and rights of all individuals, regardless of race or ethnicity, this Article contributes to the broader goal of achieving health equity and justice for Black communities.

Practical examples of a research and practice agenda for Black women that support the right to have our full humanity honored and valued include:

1. Conducting research that explores and addresses implicit biases, stereotypes, and discriminatory practices that Black women may encounter in healthcare settings. Developing interventions and training programs that promote cultural sensitivity, empathy, and respect in healthcare interactions.
2. Developing and implementing health education programs specifically tailored to the needs and experiences of Black women. These programs can provide information on self-advocacy, health literacy, and navigating the healthcare system, empowering Black women to make informed decisions about health and well-being.

3. Recognizing and addressing the intersectional experiences of Black women, such as the overlapping impacts of race, gender, socioeconomic status, and other factors on health outcomes. Incorporating an intersectional lens in research design, data collection, and analysis to better understand the unique challenges faced by Black women and develop targeted interventions.
4. Inclusive representation in research and leadership: Promoting diversity and inclusivity in research teams, healthcare organizations, and leadership positions. Ensuring that Black women are represented and have a voice in research studies, clinical trials, policy development, and decision-making processes that impact health and well-being.
5. Partnering with Black women and Black communities in the research process to co-create and implement studies that address our unique needs and priorities. Emphasizing community-based participatory research approaches that value the expertise and knowledge of Black women as active contributors and collaborators.
6. Engaging in advocacy efforts to address systemic barriers and promote policies that protect the rights and dignity of Black women. This can involve advocating for equitable access to healthcare, affordable and comprehensive health insurance coverage, anti-discrimination legislation, and eliminating health disparities.
7. Prioritizing research and practice that addresses the mental health needs of Black women, including the impact of racism, discrimination, and historical trauma. Promoting culturally sensitive and trauma-informed mental health services that support the emotional well-being of Black women.
8. Encouraging diverse and positive representations of Black women in health media and messaging. Challenging harmful stereotypes and promoting accurate portrayals highlighting the strength, resilience, and diversity of Black women's experiences.

CONCLUSION

In conclusion, this chapter has explored the Black Health Bill of Rights, a comprehensive framework that advocates for the rights and well-being of Black communities through the lens of Black women's health. Each article of the Bill of Rights highlights specific areas where significant progress is needed to achieve health equity and justice for Black people, especially Black women. From the need for a culture of health that values holistic well-being to the call for respectful and dignified healthcare, culturally sensitive approaches, and decolonized perspectives, these rights reflect the urgent need for transformative change.

Historically, Black communities have demonstrated resilience and strength in the face of systemic challenges and injustices. This chapter recognizes and celebrates this resilience while emphasizing that it should not be a justification for perpetuating health disparities. Instead, it calls for an honest acknowledgment of historical narratives and their impact on present-day health outcomes. It also emphasizes the importance of learning from the past, honoring Black heroes in health research and care, and incorporating positive aspects of African and Black American history into regular practice. Moreover, it is critical to center Black women's ways of knowing.

Furthermore, this chapter highlights the necessity of recognizing the full humanity of Black people and the ongoing struggle for equal rights. It underscores that health is a fundamental human right and emphasizes the need to address human rights issues in the context of Black health. By doing so, we harness these ontologies and epistemologies to work toward dismantling the systemic barriers that limit access to quality care, undermine well-being, and perpetuate health inequities.

Ultimately, the Black Health Bill of Rights serves as a powerful advocacy tool and a roadmap for transformative action, which is our call to action and why this book is so necessary for developing this roadmap. It calls on individuals, communities, healthcare providers, policymakers, and society as a whole to unite in the pursuit of justice, equity, and optimal health for Black people, especially Black women. By embracing the principles and values enshrined in the Bill of Rights, we can collectively create a future where every Black person is afforded the respect, dignity, and opportunities they deserve, leading to improved health outcomes and a more equitable society for all.

ABOUT THE COUNCIL ON BLACK HEALTH

The Council on Black Health is a research and action network that provides thought leadership to develop and implement a national agenda for Black health. The organization drives the agenda to realize healthy Black communities by impacting individual behaviors, social and political determinants of health, and chronic disease outcomes through a focus on partnerships, research, policy advocacy, and permanence. The Council includes academic researchers, community partners, and community leaders from across the United States who collaborate to address the variables that directly and indirectly impact Black Health. Learn more about the Council on Black Health at www.councilbh.org.

REFERENCES

Adebisi, Y. A. (2023). Decolonizing epidemiological research: A critical perspective. *Avicenna Journal of Medicine*, *13*(2), 68–76.

Airhihenbuwa, C. O., Ford, C. L., & Iwelunmor, J. I. (2014). Why culture matters in health interventions: Lessons from HIV/AIDS stigma and NCDs. *Health Education & Behavior*, *41*(1), 78–84.

Bailey, Z. D., Krieger, N., Agenor, M., Graves, J., Linos, N., & Bassett, M. T. (2017). Structural racism and health inequities in the USA: Evidence and interventions. *The Lancet*, *389*(10077), 1453–1463.

Beach, M. C., Inui, T., & Relationship-Centered Care Research Network. (2006). Relationship-centered care: A constructive reframing. *Journal of General Internal Medicine*, *21*(S1), S3–S8.

Betancourt, J. R., Green, A. R., Carrillo, J. E., & Ananeh-Firempong, O. (2003). Defining cultural competence: A practical framework for addressing racial/ethnic disparities in health and health care. *Public Health Reports*, *118*(4), 293–302. https://doi.org/10.1093/phr/118.4.293

Chandra, A., Acosta, J., Carman, K. G., Dubowitz, T., Leviton, L., Martin, L. T., Miller, C., Nelson, C., Orleans, T., Tait, M., Trujillo, M., Towe, V., Yeung, D., & Plough, A. L. (2017). Building a national culture of health: Background, action framework, measures, and next steps. *Rand Health Q*, *6*(2), 3. 28845341.

Chinn, J. J., Martin, I. K., & Redmond, N. (2021). Health equity among Black women in the United States. *Journal of Women's Health*, *30*(2), 212–219. https://doi.org/10.1089/jwh.2020.8868

Crear-Perry, J., Maybank, A., Keeys, M., Mitchell, N., & Godbolt, D. (2020). Moving towards anti-racist praxis in medicine. *The Lancet*, *396*(10249), 451–453.

Crenshaw, K. (1989). Demarginalizing the intersection of race and sex: A black feminist critique of antidiscrimination doctrine, feminist theory and antiracist politics. *University of Chicago Legal Forum*, *1*(8), 139–167.

Czyzewski, K. (2011). Colonialism as a broader social determinant of health. *The International Indigenous Policy Journal*, *2*(1), 5.

Davis, A. Y. (2005). *Abolition Democracy: Beyond Empire, Prisons, and Torture*. Seven Stories Press.

DeSantis, C. E., Miller, K. D., Sauer, A. G., Jemal, A., & Siegel, R. L. (2019). Cancer statistics for African Americans, 2019. *CA: A Cancer Journal for Clinicians*, *69*(3), 211–233. https://doi.org/10.3322/caac.21555

Dyrbye, L. N., Thomas, M. R., & Shanafelt, T. D. (2006). Systematic review of depression, anxiety, and other indicators of psychological distress among U.S. and Canadian medical students. *Academic Medicine*, *81*(4), 354–373.

Fiscella, K., & Sanders, M. R. (2016). Racial and ethnic disparities in the quality of health care. *Annual Review of Public Health*, *37*, 375–394.

Foronda, C., Baptiste, D.-L., Reinholdt, M. M., & Ousman, K. (2016). Cultural humility: A concept analysis. *Journal of Transcultural Nursing*, *27*(3), 210–217. https://doi.org/10.1177/1043659615592677

Gamble, V. N. (1997). Under the shadow of Tuskegee: African Americans and health care. *American Journal of Public Health*, *87*(11), 1773–1778.
Huber, M., Knottnerus, J. A., Green, L., Horst, H. v., Jadad, A. R., & Kromhout, D. (2011). How should we define health? *BMJ*, *34*, 1–33.
Minehart, R. D., Bryant, A. S., Jackson, J., & Daly, J. L. (2021). Racial/ethnic inequities in pregnancy-related morbidity and mortality. *Obstetrics and Gynecology Clinics of North America*, *48*(1), 31–51.
National Center for Health Statistics. (2023). *Health, United States, 2020–2021: Annual Perspective*. Hyattsville, MD. Retrieved July, 2023, from https://stacks.cdc.gov/view/cdc/122044
Paradies, Y. (2006). A systematic review of empirical research on self-reported racism and health. *International Journal of Epidemiology*, *35*(4), 888–901.
Peters, S. A., Huxley, R. R., & Woodward, M. (2014). Diabetes as a risk factor for stroke in women compared with men: A systematic review and meta-analysis of 64 cohorts, including 775,385 individuals and 12,539 strokes. *The Lancet*, *383*(9933), 1973–1980. https://doi.org/10.1016/S0140-6736(14)60040-4
Petersen, E. E., Davis, N. L., Goodman, D., Cox, S., Syverson, C., Seed, K., Shapiro-Mendoza, C., Callaghan, W. M., & Barfield, W. (2019). Racial/ethnic disparities in pregnancy-related deaths — United States, 2007–2016. *Morbidity and Mortality Weekly Report*, *68*(35), 762–765. https://doi.org/10.15585/mmwr.mm6835a3
Ryan, R. M., & Deci, E. L. (2000). Self-determination theory and the facilitation of intrinsic motivation, social development, and well-being. *American Psychologist*, *55*(1), 68–78. https://psycnet.apa.org/doi/10.1037/0003-066X.55.1.68
Sekaquaptewa, D., Waldman, A., & Thompson, M. (2007). Solo status and self-construal: Being distinctive influences racial self-construal and performance apprehension in African American women. *Cultural Diversity & Ethnic Minority Psychology*, *13*(4), 321–327. https://doi.org/10.1037/1099-9809.13.4.321
Sium, A., Desai, C., & Ritskes, E. (2012). Towards the 'tangible unknown': Decolonization and the indigenous future. *Decolonization, Indigeneity, Education, & Society*, *1*(1), I–XIII.
Triandis, H. C. (2018). *Individualism and Collectivism*. Taylor & Francis Group.
Utsey, S. O., Giesbrecht, N., Hook, J., & Stanard, P. M. (2008). Cultural, sociofamilial, and psychological resources that inhibit psychological distress in African Americans exposed to stressful life events and race-related stress. *Journal of Counseling Psychology*, *55*(1), 49–62.
Williams, D. R., & Mohammed, S. A. (2013). Racism and health I: Pathways and scientific evidence. *American Behavioral Scientist, 57*(8), 1152–1173.

Index

ableism, 156
abolition, 43, 50, 52
abortion, 4–5; bans, 50; funds, 50; protections, 51
abuse, 15, 62; academic, 71; in Black communities, 45; of Black women, 18; emotional, 46; neglect and, 101; racial-gendered, 68; systematic, 68
accessibility, 104, 160, 190
active listening, 119
activism, 5, 8, 24, 105, 117; movement, 57
Adams, Alma, 176
Adams, Jerome, 168
Adichie, Chimamanda, 187
adverse health outcomes, 5
advocacy, 117, 219
affirmative action, 51, 60
Affuso, Olivia, 11, 201
African American Vernacular English, 139
African ascent, 31
African descent, 31
African Diaspora, 31, 131, 170, 191
aggressions, 86–87
alcohol, 22
alcoholism, 167
allostatic load, 16
allyship, 5
AMA. *See* American Medical Association (AMA)
American English, 139
American Medical Association (AMA), 171
American Psychological Association, 134
American Revolution, 1
Amutah-Onukagha, Ndidi, 171
ancestral knowledge, 2
Anderson, Brittany N., 152
angry Black woman stereotype, 96
Anti-Defamation League, 20
Anti-Defamation League Center on Extremism (COE), 60
Anti-Racists Pedagogy, 153
anti-Semitism, 156
anxiety, 49, 139, 143–44
Anything We Love Can be Saved, 46
Anzaldúa, Gloria, 168
Arango Ricks, Shawn, 11, 95–106
arts-based approach, 81–82
Association for the Study of African American Life and History (ASALH), 87
Association of Black Psychologists, 134
asthma, 49
autonomy, bodily, 1, 4–5, 159–60, 213–15

Avery, Byllye Y., 5, 176

Baartman, Saartjie, 86
Bailey, Moya, 5
Bailey, Zinzi D., 148
The Balanced Black Girl podcast, 87
Bambara, Toni Cade, 31, 54–55
Barlow, Jameta Nicole, 1–11, *3*, 35, 53, 87, 171, 201
Becton, Dajerria, 20
behavior, destructive, 95
Berger, Michelle T., 3
Between Good & Ghetto, 35
"Beyond the Side Eye," 71
BFW. *See* Black Feminist and Womanist (BFW) Analytical Path to Health Equity
BGWH. *See* Black girls' and women's health (BGWH)
bias, 60, 135, 178; identify and address, 119; implicit, 111, 167, 207–14; individual, 65; medical, 197; provider, 17–18, 206; racial, 176
bi-directional mentoring, 36
Big Momma, 168–74
birthworkers, 3, 5, 8
Black churches, 20
Black culture, 46
Black Diaspora, 188
Black educators, in sex education, 157–58
Black Feminism(s): canon, 34; ethnography, 35–36; health science, 5; ideals, 2, 6–10, 35, 44–47, 90, 191; legacy of, 8; movements, 45; praxis, 34; principles, 90; theories, 58; theorists, 45
Black Feminism-as-action, 35
Black Feminism Thought, 105, 153
Black Feminist and Womanist (BFW) Analytical Path to Health Equity, 2
Black Feminist and Womanist Thought, 10
Black Feminist Consciousness, 8, 10, 44
Black Feminist Hauntology, 71
Black Feminist legal theory, 6
Black Feminist Ontologies, 9
Black Feminist Studies, 10
Black Feminist Thought, 155
Black Feminist Thought, 59
Black Femmes, 62–65
Black folx, 5
Black futures, 6
Blackgirl, 31; communities, 32; epistemologies, 33; health, 40; health science, 1–11, *3*; lived experiences of, 3; methodology, 37; urban, 35; voices, 109–14, *115*, 116–20; wellness praxis, 39–40
Black Girlhood, 32–33
"Black Girl Magic," 32, 116
Black girls' and women's health (BGWH), 194–96; interdisciplinary and transdisciplinary approaches to, 2; philosophy, 6–7; reclaiming of, 8–10
Black Girls' and Women's Health Research and Praxis Collaborative, 2
A Black Girl's Guide to Weight Loss, 176
Blackgirls' health science, philosophy of, 1–11, *3*
Black Girls Run, 86
Blackgirl wellness: praxis of, 36, 39–40; ways of being, 32; ways of documenting, 37–39; ways of doing, 36–37; ways of knowing, 33–36; words and, 31–32
Black health, reimagining of, 203–19
Black Health Bill of Rights, 11, 203, 219; right to culture of health that values well-being, 204–6; right to have humanity honored and valued, 217–18; right to honor past, present, and future, 215–16; right to power and autonomy, 213–15; right to receive culturally sensitive care, 208–10; right to receive respectful and dignified healthcare, 206–8; right to strengths-based approach to health equity, 211–13

Black joy, 159–61
Black Lives Matter, 177
Black Macho and the Myth of the Superwoman, 95
Black Mamas Matter Alliance, 171, 176
Black Maternal Health Caucus, 176
Black Maternal Health Momnibus Act of 2020, 176
Black Maternal Health Research Re-Envisioned, 176
Black movements, 105
Black mysticisms, 6
Black Nationalism, 105
Blackness, 156
Black people, 1
Black Power movement, 45–46
Black Queer Feminism, 63–65
Black reading, to heal, 52–55
"Black Reading to Heal," 52–55
Black reproductive justice, 6
Black resistance, 50
Blackstock, Uche, 22
Black trans women, 63–64
Black Woman ethos, 79
Black Womanism, 45; working-class, 57. *See also* Womanism(s)
Black women: empowerment of, 8; health, 15–17; way forward for, 24–26; at work, 23–24
Black Women and Self Recovery, 48
Black Women's Health: future of, 21–22; implications for, 21; utility of love for, 43–55
Black Women's Health Imperative, 5, 15, 176
Black Women's Health Study, 16–17
Black writings, 48
Bland, Sandra, 43
bodily autonomy, 1, 4–5
body: image, 135; positivity, 160–61
books, banned, 55, 156
Boston, Asha, 177
Boston Black Women's Health Study, 5
Boylorn, Robin, 31
Brathwaite, Brittany, 36
breakdown, breakthrough and, 97–101
The Bridge Called My Back, 168
Brown, Ruth Nicole, 35
Browne, Mahogany L., 32, 39
Brown James, Lexx, 160
Burford, Tanisha, 128
Burke, Tarana, 177
burnout: or stress, 101–2; symptoms, 100
Burst of Light, 106

Callier, Shawneequa, 171
cancer, 17, 70, 167, 201; breast, 18, 22, 49
"The Cancer Journals," 49
"Can Watching Racist Viral Videos Give You PTSD?," 20
capitalism, 3, 52, 104
cardiovascular disease, 17, 143–44
career status, in workplace, 142
Carr, Greg, 4
CBPR. *See* community-based participatory research (CBPR)
Celebrating Twenty Years of Black Girlhood, 175
Christianity, 1, 78
chronic disease, 178, 201, 217
Church Terrell, Mary, 8
citationality, 61
civil rights activism, 24
clinical research practice, 16
COE. *See* Anti-Defamation League Center on Extremism (COE)
collaborative care, 119
collective freedom, 89
collective spaces, 91
collective spirit, 79
collectivism, 205
colonialism, 7, 124
colonial masculinity, 62
colonization, 211
colonizing language, 4
color-blind ideology, 109
colorism, 141–42
The Color Purple, 46

Combahee Feminist Collective, 9
Combahee River Collective, 7, 45, 188
communication, 1, 77–78; culturally responsive, 119
communities: Black, 5–6; Blackgirl, 32; LGBTQIA+, 51, 63, 79; organizations, 208; praxis, 44, 167–69, 174–77; relationships in, 125; vernacular, 4
community-based participatory research (CBPR), 124, 212
compartmentalization, of Blackgirls' lives, 31
concrete ceiling, breaking of, 139–44
confidence, 85
conformation, 85–86
constructivism, 126–27
content creators, 5
contraception, 151
contributions, erasure of, 62
Cooper, Anna Julia, 7–8, 45
coping: mechanisms, 98–100, 113; skills, 105; strategies, *115*, 118, 139
cortisol, 16, 69
Council on Black Health, 201, 217
Crear-Perry, Joia Adele, 168, 171
Creating A Respectful and Open World for Natural Hair (CROWN) Act, 135–36, 140
Crenshaw, Kimberlé, 59, 155, 177, 179
Critical Race Feminism, 105
Critical Race Theory (CRT), 7, 105, 178
critical reflexivity, 83
critical social theories, 105
CROWN. *See* Creating A Respectful and Open World for Natural Hair (CROWN) Act
CRT. *See* Critical Race Theory (CRT)
Cullors, Patrisse, 177
cultural humility, 208–10
culturally responsive health praxis, Blackgirls' voices in, 109, 120; framework for, 111–14, *115*, 116–17; reimagination of, 117–19; science philosophy in, 110
culture, 4, 61, 88, 154; African, 131; Black, 46, 114, 144, 151; capitalistic, 170; expression of, 1; of health, 204–6; white dominant, 38, 139; in workplace, 23

The Danger of a Single Story, 187
Davis, Angela, 103, 190
death, premature, 22
decolonial psychology, 58
decolonization, 62, 211–13; healing and, 70–72; process of, 67
Decolonizing Methodologies, 61
"defund the police," 50
depression, 44, 49, 100, 139, 143–44
Devoe, Y. Falami, 11, 23, 77–91
dexamethasone, 18
diabetes, 17, 22, 49, 143, 201
Dickens, Danielle, 11, 22, 139–44
Dill, LeConté J., 10, 25, 31–40, 174
Dinnertable Documentary, 177
discrimination, 65, 116, 136, 175–77, 205–8, 218; experiences of, 60, 139–42; forms of, 201, 203–5, 209–12; gender, 16–23, 26, 47, 52; racial, 148; in workplace, 139
disposability, 44, 50
Dixon, Morgan, 176
Dixon Diallo, Dázon, 172
double consciousness, 78
doulas, 5, 50, 176, 223
DuBois, W. E. B., 78, 135, 190
Dunn, Mercedez, 36

Ebony, 135
economic oppression, 19
educational system, violent history of, 58
Emanuel African Methodist Episcopal Church, 20
empathy, 9, 25, 39, 119
Enacting Our Multidimensional Power, 153
epistemologies, 2, *3*, 17, 71, 211; ancestral, 4; Blackgirl, 33; Feminist, 110, 188; Womanist, 10, 80, 188

equality, 63, 217; intersectional, 10; struggle for, 9
equity, 188; health, 2, 19–21, 169, 171, 189, 204–19, 224; structural, 208–10
erasure, 3, 34, 61–62, 147, 155–57
Evans, Stephanie, 6
Evans-Winters, Venus, 6, 64, 168, 172
Everything But The Kitchen Sink, 23

Family and Medical Leave Act (FMLA), 100
Fanon, Frantz, 135
Feminism, 110, 156; Black, 2, 6, 8–10, 35–36, 44–47, 90, 191; critical race, 105; white, 157
feminist movement, second wave, 8
Feminist Theory, 105
Femme, 62; sex educators, 147. *See also* Black femmes
femmes women of color, 5
Fields, Jessica, 150
Flowers, Sara, 11, 25, 147–61, *154*
Floyd, George, 20, 50, 171
FMLA. *See* Family and Medical Leave Act (FMLA)
Fullilove, Mindy, 173

GA. *See* "The Guided Autobiography" (GA)
Garofolo, Juliette, 188–89, 195
Garrison, Vanessa, 176
Gary-Smith, Mariotta, 160
Garza, Alicia, 177
gender: binary, 62; discrimination, 16–23, 26, 47, 52; interrogations, 6; marginalized, 51; non-conforming, 63; violence, 38
gendered racial microaggressions, 60
gendered racism, 95, 102, 116
genocide, 7
Geronimus, Arline, 16
GHA. *See* Guided Hair Autobiography (GHA)
Gilbert, Tracie, Q., 160
Girl Trek, 176
Glover, S. T., 66–70
Goler Blount, Linda, 5, 10, 15–26
GRA. *See* The Guided Race Autobiography (GRA)
granny midwives, 5
"The Guided Autobiography" (GA), 127
Guided Hair Autobiography (GHA), 128, 135–36
guided hair autobiography, as health assessment, 123–24; curriculum for, 133–36; development of, 127–29; hair, health, and heritage study in, 129–30; hair historian and, 130–32; hair school and, 132–33; unconventional constructivist and, 125–27
"The Guided Race Autobiography" (GRA), 128
Gumbs, Alexis Pauline, 70
Guy-Sheftall, Beverly, 9, 173

hair: care, 133; criminalization of, 140; CROWN, 135–36; culture and history of, 130; health, heritage and, 129–30; historian, 130–32; mental healthcare and, 133–36; natural, 136; rituals, 131; school, 132–33; stereotypes, 133; trauma, 131; workplace and, 140–41
Hair, Health, and Heritage Study, 129–30
"Hair story," 130
Hamer, Fannie Lou, 187
Hannah-Jones, Nicole, 155
harassment, 89
Harden Bradford, Joy, 176
Harlins, Latasha, 34
Harper, Frances E. W., 8
Harris, Kamala, 176
hate crimes, 20, 60
Hayes, Christie, 175
Hayward Cooper, Anna Julia, 8
HBCU. *See* Historically Black College (HBCU)
health: behaviors, 3; definition of, 15–17; disparities, 24, 99, 110, 149;

equity, 20, 211–13; establishment, 4; implications, 57–72; interventions, 109; meaning of, 15; outcomes, 109; promotion, 109
healthcare: culturally sensitive, 208–10; industry, 49, 208–10; outcomes, 118; providers, 111; reimagination of, 120; respectful and dignified, 206–8; services, underutilization of, 111; traditional approaches to, 111
health science: for Blackgirls, 1–11, *3*; healing within, 70–72; inquiry, 111; intervention, 5–8; philosophy of, 2–4, *3*; powerful words in, 2; re-claiming of, 8–10; women's, 1–11, *3*; written path in, 4–5
heart disease, 22
Heckler, Margaret, 24
Henry, Velma, 31
Hersey, Tricia, 104, 168
heteronormativity, 79
Hill, Dominique C., 31
Hill Collins, Patricia, 9, 45, 58, 80, 105, 155, 174
Hip hop, 96
historical exclusion, of Black communities, 6
Historically Black College (HBCU), 24, 110
historical oppression, 17
historical trauma, epigenetic effects of, 17
history, 1, 215–16
HIV, 18, 151
holistic health intervention, 118–19, 218
homecoming, *3*
homophobia, 69, 156
Hood Feminism, 156
hooks, bell, 44–48, 51–54, 68, 103, 168, 174
How I Stopped Playing the Strong Black Woman, 95
How It Feels to Be Colored Me, 191
humanity: honored and valued, 217–18; loss of, 1
Hurt, Byron, 96
hypertension, 143, 201

identity politics, 7
identity shifting, 139–40, 143–44
Ignace, Veroneque, 36
imagination, 1, 22
implicit bias, 111, 167, 207–14
incarceration, rates of, 116
inclusion, 160
Indigenous, 65
infant mortality, 17
inflammatory response, 17
In Lifting As I Climb, Resting When I Need, 24
In Search of Our Mothers' Garden, 47
intergenerational fatigue, 175
intersectionality, 7, 47, 179; concept of, 59
intervention, 5–8
"Invisibility Blues," 68
Isaac, Carlysha, 188, 190, 197

Jackson, Imani, 141
James, Joy, 45
Jernigan-Noesi, Maryam M., 11, 22, 109–14, *115*, 116–20
jezebel stereotype, 95–96
Johnson, Breya, 10, 25, 43–55, 186, 192–93, 198
Jones, Camara Phyllis, 24, 171
Jones, Nikki, 35
Jordan, June, 70, 173
Jordan, Valin, 174
Jordan-Zachery, Julia S., 71
Junious, Toni, 186–87, 192–94, 197–98
justice, 25, 219; fight for, 171–72; reproductive, 43
juvenile courts, 116

Kakooza, Martha, 187, 190–92
KAVI. *See* Kings Against Violence Initiative (KAVI)
Kendall, Erika Nicole, 176
Kendall, Mikki, 156–57

Kings Against Violence Initiative (KAVI), 38–39
Kinloch, Valerie, 173
kitchen table, 77–78, 87, 90–91
knowledge: ancestral, 2; apartheid, 172; of black femmes, 58–59; development of, 2; producers, 57–58; situated, 112; spiritual, 2; system, 3
knubia, 4
Kumanyika, Shiriki, 11, 201

Lachè Sutton, Shaleah, 177
Ladson-Billings, Gloria, 173
land theft, 7
language, 44; African American Vernacular English, 139; American English, 139; colonizing, 4; control of, 1; native, 1; as thought and action, 1
Laureano, Bianca I., 160
Lee Alves, Cindy, 160
legal system, criminal, 36
Lewis, Tené, 16
Lewis-Ragland, Yolanda, 172
LGBTQIA+ community, 79; protections, 51; safeguards for, 63
liberation, 1, 160; of American Black women, 8; of Black people, 4; fight for, 57; movements, 43
Lifting as We Climb, 95; breakdown and breakthrough, 97–101; rest and, 103–4; science philosophy and, 105–6; silencing and, 96–97; stress or burnout, 101–2; trauma definition and, 102–3
light skin privilege, 141
Listen to Black Women, 176
lived experiences, of Black Women, 77; aggressions and, 86–87; arts-based approaches, 81, 82; arts-based researcher, 81–82; call to action and, 90–91; conforming and, 85–86; foundation of, 83; reimagining and, 87–90; Sankofa, 83; science philosophy, 78–79; Womanism and, 79–81
The Look of Love, 46
Lorde, Audre, 45, 49, 70, 86, 103–6, 150, 179
love: politics, 45–48; radical, 45–48, 52; utility of, 43–55
Love, Bettina, 37
lupus, 49

madea, 170
Mallory, Tamika, 173
mammy stereotype, 95–96, 168
Maparyan, Layli (Phillips), 10, 79–80
marginalization, 96; double, 139
Martin, Trayvon, 43
maternal mortality, 17, 22
Mbilishaka, Afiya, 11, 22, 123–36
McAdams, Dan, 127
McGoy, Shanell, 177
McKittrick, Katherine, 59
McLeod Bethune, Mary, 8
Media Psychology Review, 135
medical school, 171
medicines, natural, 57
memories, 127
Mendez, Dara, 171
mental distress, 87
mental healthcare, 51–52, 95; evaluation, 105; hair and, 123, 133–36; services, 123; stigma and, 102, 126, 133
Mental Health Facts for African Americans, 51
Mental Health First Aid (MHFA), 133
meritocracy, 25
methodology, *3*; decolonizing, 7
Me Too, 177
MHFA. *See* Mental Health First Aid (MHFA)
midwives, 3–4, 8; granny, 5
minority, 21
misogyny, 58, 69, 149–50, 156
Moore, Susan, 18
Morago, Cherrie, 168
Morris, Monique, 173
Morrison, Toni, 6–7, 10, 44–48, 147, 159, 188

movement activism, 57
Multidimensional Power framework, 153, *154*, 155

NACW. *See* National Association for Colored Women (NACW)
names, 1
The Nap Ministry, 103, 168, 173
Narrative Photovoice, 87
narratives, embodied, 57–72
Nash, Jennifer, 45, 47
Nathani Wane, Njoki, 170
National Association for Colored Women (NACW), 96
National Birth Equity Collaborative, 171
National Institutes of Health (NIH), 19
National Women's Studies Association (NWSA), 101
Nat Turner Rebellion, 1
Neale Hurston, Zora, 7, 191
Nelly, 96
Newport, Cal, 125
NIH. *See* National Institutes of Health (NIH)
non-binary, 63; students, 65
normalized chaos, 97
NWSA. *See* National Women's Studies Association (NWSA)

Obama, Barack, 20
obesity, 17, 38, 143, 201
Occam's razor, 104
Okafor, Chinyere, 10–11, 22, 57–72
ontologies, 2, *3*, 17
opioids, 18
oppression, 105; racial, 143; in research and clinical practice, 123; resistance to, 8, 116–17; systemic, 110; systems of, 156
other-mothering, as community praxis, 167–79
Out of Racism, The Scholar, 15–26

pain: dismissal of, 111; tolerance, 151
pain medication, 18
Parks, Rosa, 6
participatory action research project, 87–88
participatory narrative analysis, 37
patient-centered care, 119
patriarchy, 3, 44; of academy, 24
"pedagogy of disposability," 44
Pedagogy of the Oppressed, 71
Peoples, Whitney, 5
perspective, 1
"Pet to Threat," 23, 142
philosophy: of Blackgirls' health science, 1–11, *3*; science, 110; of science, 2, 43, 61–62, 78–79, 105–6; of women's health science, 1–11, *3*
photography, 82
PhotoNovella, 88
PhotoVoice, 89–90; methodology, 82
Pierce, Chester, 59
Pinckney, Clementa C., 20
Pintor Carnagey, Melissa, 160
Planet Venus, 172
police: Black deaths from, 20; brutality, 50; defund, 50
policy, 16, 19; advocacy, 216; analysis, 9; briefs, 37; makers, 20; unspoken, 102
political movement, 10
politics: identity, 7; love, 45–48; Queer, 89; racial, 69; resistance in, 55; sexual, 69; tension in, 50
positionality, in workplace, 140
power, 213–15
Practicing Love, 47
praxis, 6, 19, 26, 118, 120; of Blackgirl wellness, 39–40; community, 44, 167–79; healing, 48–52
predominantly white institutions (PWIs), 66, 99–100, 185–86
pregnancy, 4–5, 151
Presumed Incompetent, 59
Promising Futures, 174, 177
provider bias care, 17–18, 206
psychoanalysis, 43

PsychoHairapist, 133
PsychoHairapy, 87, 123; certification, 134; Research Lab, 128
psychology, 2; Black, 43; of hair, 129
PsychoTherapy space, 87
PTSD, 49
public health, 2, 16; practice, 21, 32; reimagination of, 31; theory, 32
PWIs. *See* predominantly white institutions (PWIs)

Queer theory, 58

RA. *See* resident assistant (RA)
race narratives, 127; therapy, 128
Race Self Complexity, 127
racial differences, denial of, 109
racial microaggressions, 59; gendered, 60
racial socialization, 134
racism, 114; black embodiment and, 59–61; in education, 140; expectations, 22; function of, 6; gendered, 95, 102, 116; institutional, 149; internalized, 24; medical, 149; out of, 15–26; scientific, 67; structural, 148, 156, 167; systemic, 124, 149; in workplace, 23
radical humanism, 45
radicalization, 43
radical love, 45–48, 52
Ransom, Minnie, 31
reading, illegal, 1
Re-Imagining Black Girls' and Women's Health Symposium and Workshop, 2
religions, traditional, 1
representation, lack of, 111, 124
reproductive care, 50
reproductive justice, 43
research, 6, 21–22, 26; academic health, 124, 219; art-informed, 81; arts-based, 81–82; Black, 19; CBPR, 124; clinical, 19; community-accountable, 37; development, 5; funding for, 19; gender, 112; interdisciplinary, 140; methods class, 125; participatory action, 87; process, 126; psychology, 124; race-neutral, 178; scientists, 126; social, 19; social science, 62; studies, 90
resident assistant (RA), 192
resilience, 114, *115*, 116, 215
resistance, 114, *115*, 116, 117
rest, 95, 103–4
"Rest is Resistance" framework, 104
Ricks, Shawn Arango, 24
right-wing fascism, 60
rituals, 33, 37; hair, 131; spiritual, 136
Roberts, Dorothy, 171
Robert Wood Johnson Foundation, 204
Roe v. Wade, 50
'Rona. *See* SARS-COV2/COVID19 pandemic
Rose, Tricia, 174
Rowley, Diane, 171
rules, unspoken, 97

safety, 38
The Salt Eaters, 31, 54
sameness, emphasis on, 109
Sankofa, 83–85
SARS-COV2/COVID19 pandemic, 4, 18–19, 51, 70, 167, 173, 175
Saving Our Lives Hear Our Truths (SOLHOT), 33, 35
SayHerName, 177
SBW. *See* Strong Black Woman (SBW)
science: philosophy, 2–4, *3*, 43, 61–62, 78–79, 105–6, 110; social, 62
Scott, Trina, 160
self-actualization, 189
self-care, 9–10, 25, 100, 103, 105
self-concept, 113, 152
self-esteem, 152
self-love, 45, 100–101, 103
self-medication, 22
self-preservation, 25
self-recovery, 53
self-regulation, 106

settler colonial project, 65
sex education: accessibility and, 160; Black educators in, 157–58; Black joy and, 159–61; body positivity and, 160–61; context in, 149–52; curriculum, 151, 157, 159; evolution of, 159; program development, 158; solutions for, 152–57, *154*; white ethnocentricity and, 148; white gaze and, 147–48
sexism, 68, 114, 124; in education, 140
Sex Positive Families, 160
sexual health, 148
sexually transmitted infections (STIs), 150, 159
sexual violence, 38, 87
Shakur, Assata, 45
Shange, Ntozake, 45
Shaull, Richard, 71
Sheats, Jylana, 177
sickle cell disease, 18–19
silencing, 96–97
Simone, Nina, 45–46
Simpson, Georgina Rose, 57
Sisters of the Yam, 48, 53, 168
situational awareness, social constructivist theory and, 154–55
The 1619 Project, 156
slave: owners, 4; plantations, 66; states, 1
slavery, 102, 104, 147, 211; Africa, 7; institution of, 1
Smith, Olivia, 175
social activists, 8
social constructivist theory, situational awareness and, 154–55
social determinants of health, 109, *115*, 151, 175, 205–19
social justice: projects, 105; teaching praxis, 175
social listening, 16
societal norms, 140
SOLHOT. *See* Saving Our Lives Hear Our Truths (SOLHOT)
The Souls of Black Folk, 78
Southampton Insurrection, 1
Southern Black Feminisms Health Framework, 2
Southern Medical Journal, 4
Speaking for Ourselves, 174
spirit murder, 66
spiritual healthcare, 136
spiritual knowledge, 2
spiritual practices, traditional, 1
spiritual rituals, 136
Stalter, Madelyn, 188–89, 195–96
Standpoint Theory, 105
Stanley-Jones, Aiyana, 43
stereotypes, 86, 95, 119, 147, 150, 155; gender, 113–14; hair, 133; harmful, 124; pressure from, 97; racial, 113–14
Stevenson, Tambra, 11, 176, 201
Stewart, Maria, 8
stigma, 102, 126; mental healthcare and, 133
STIs. *See* sexually transmitted infections (STIs)
stories, health implications of: black femmes, 58–59; Black Queer Feminist lens, 63–65; Black women as knowledge producers in, 57–58; counternarratives and, 67–70; decolonization and, 70–72; educational system violence, 58; health sciences and, 70–72; racism and black embodiment, 59–61; science philosophy, 61–62; settler colonial project, 65; spirit murder, 66; survival pedagogies, 66–67; university violence, 65
stories, of lived experiences, 77–91
storytelling, power of, 67–70
strengths-based approach, 211–13
stress, 44, 69; burnout or, 101–2; chronic, 98–100; internalized, 106; persistent, 16; in workplace, 139–44; workplace and, 143–44
stroke, 22
Strong Black Woman (SBW), 102, 196; stereotype, 95–96

structural determinants of health, 176
structural oppression, 3
structural racism, 148; background, 169–70; Big Mommas work, 171–74; community praxis and, 174–77; government and, 177–79; science philosophy, 167–69
substance misuse, 22
suicide, 52
Superwoman Schema, 174
survival, pedagogies of, 66–67
Sutton, Shavaun, 36

"Talking Back," 68
Tarika Art, 3
Taylor, Breonna, 20, 50, 171
Theory for Liberatory Practice, 53
Theory of gender and power, 153–54
Therapy for Black Girls, 87, 176
A Third University is Possible, 65
tokenism, 67, 98, 139, 155
Tometi, Opal, 177
Townsend, Shanna-Kay, 36
TransAtlantic Slave Trade, 1–2
transgender, 63; college students, 65; women of color, 5, 10
transmisogynoir, 63
transphobia, 63, 156
trauma, 38, 104, 144; definition, 102–3; hair, 131; historical, 111; inherited, 52; racial, 104
Truth, Sojourner, 8
Tuhiwai, Linda, 61

Underwood, Lauren, 176
Uniquely You Summit, 177

vernacular, communities', 4
violence, 20; academic institutional, 59; administrative, 65; in education system, 58; epistemic, 36; gender, 38; from healthcare providers, 50; indirect, 70; institutional, 66; KAVI, 38–39; management strategies, 38; against marginalized genders, 51; physical, 80; prevention, 38; relationship, 90; sexual, 38, 87; systemic, 80; of university, 65; against women, 51

Walker, Alice, 45–47, 79, 103, 188
Wallace, Michele, 68–69, 95
WANDA. *See* Women Advancing Nutrition, Dietetics, and Agriculture (WANDA)
Ward, Maranda, 11, 25, 167–79
weathering, 16
weight gain, 17, 100
well-being, 205; valued, 204
wellness, experiences of, 31. *See also* Blackgirl wellness
Wells Barnett, Ida B., 8
white dominant culture, 139
white ethnocentricity, 147–48, 152, 159; subconscious, 149
white gaze, 148–49, 151, 159; impact of, 147
whiteness, 3
white savior complex, 149
white supremacy, 7, 34, 44, 155; propaganda, 60
Whitt-Glover, Melicia, 11, 201
Whyte, Danielle, 187, 189–90, 193, 196
Williams, Serena, 207
Winston-Proctor, Cynthia, 128
WISH. *See* Women, Intersectionality, Science, and Health (WISH) Writing Lab; Women In Science and Health (WISH)
withdrawal, 114, *115*
WoCSHN. *See* Women of Color Sexual Health Network (WoCSHN)
Womanism(s), 80–81; African, 125; Africana, 136; epistemologies, 10; health science, 1–11, *3*; ideology of, 110; methodologies, 10; perspective, 78; scholar, 78–79
Womanist: proclamation of, 80; scholar, 43

Women, Intersectionality, Science, and Health (WISH) Writing Lab: change and, 185–86; positionality, 189–93; possibilities for, 198–99; reasons for, 186–89; unique gifts for, 193–98
Women Advancing Nutrition, Dietetics, and Agriculture (WANDA), 176
Women In Science and Health (WISH), 11, 22
Women of Color Sexual Health Network (WoCSHN), 160
Woods Giscombé, Cheryl, 174
words, power of, 2
workplace, Black women in, 139; authenticity in, 144; career status and shifting in, 142; colorism in, 141–42; hair and shifting in, 140–41; positionality in, 140; stress and identity shifting in, 143–44
workplace culture, 23
writing, illegal, 1
written path, 4–5
written word, 4–5; power of, 1

About the Editor

Jameta Nicole Barlow, *PhD, MPH, The George Washington University*

Jameta Nicole Barlow, PhD, MPH, RYT® 200, a Charlottesville, Virginia native, is a community psychologist, women's health scholar and an assistant professor of writing in The George Washington University's University Writing Program and Women's Leadership Program. She holds secondary appointments in the Women's, Gender & Sexuality Studies Program in the Columbian College of Arts and Sciences and the Department of Health Policy and Management in the Milken Institute of Public Health. She is also an affiliate faculty member in the Global Women's Institute, Africana Studies Program and the Jacobs Institute of Women's Health. Dr. Barlow is the Director of Undergraduate Studies for the Women's, Gender & Sexuality Studies Program. Her research utilizes decolonizing methodologies to disrupt cardiometabolic syndrome and structural policies adversely affecting Black girls' and women's health, intergenerational trauma, and perinatal mental health. Dr. Barlow uses Black Feminisms and Womanism to theorize, implement, and evaluate methodologies, interventions, and policies for Black girls and women. With professional experiences in federal government, national non-profits and academia, she has spent 24 years in transdisciplinary collaborations with physicians, public health practitioners, researchers, policy administrators, activists, political appointees, and community members in diverse settings throughout the world. Certified as an Emotional Emancipation Circle Facilitator and vinyasa and restorative yoga instructor, Dr. Barlow is also trained as a doula, childbirth educator, and prenatal yoga and meditation instructor; and, a 2015 AcademyHealth/Aetna Foundation Scholar-in-Residence Fellow, 2016 RAND Faculty Leaders Fellow in Policy Research and Analysis, and 2020–2021 GW Humanities Center Fellow. Dr. Barlow has served in a variety of leadership roles within the American Psychological Association, including the American Psychological Association of Graduate Students and as the Immediate Past Chair for the American Psychological Association's Committee on Women in Psychology. Additionally, she is the inaugural Scholar-in-Residence at the Black Women's Health Imperative and Strategic Communications and Implementation Advisor for the Council on Black Health.

A 2023 Public Voices Fellowship at AcademyHealth, in partnership with The OpEd Project, Dr. Barlow's writings on Black girls' and women's health, intersectionality, health equity, healing, and restorative health practices in psychology and public health research appear in various publications and she offers community-based and industry focused workshops and trainings on these topics. Dr. Barlow has been quoted in *The New York Times*, *The Washington Post*, *Essence*, *Shape*, *Insider*, *NBC News*, *OZY*, *mashable*, *the Skimm*, *Medical News Today*, *NPR*, *Psych Central*, and *Healthline*. She presents her work in various forms of media. Her digital storytelling work, the Saving Our Sisters Project (www.savingoursistersproject.com), is focused on Black women's mental health and well-being, employing writing and the personal narrative. She believes her evidence-based curriculum, "writehealing," is an effective approach towards uncovering trauma and healing. Dr. Barlow holds a Bachelor of Arts (BA) in English from Spelman College, a Master of Public Health (MPH) in Maternal and Child Health from The George Washington University, and a Doctor of Philosophy (PhD) in Psychology from North Carolina State University.

About the Contributors

Olivia Affuso, *PhD, FACSM; Director, Strategic Leadership Initiatives; Council on Black Health*

Dr. Olivia Affuso, FACSM is the newly appointed Director of Strategic Leadership Initiatives at the Council on Black Health, formerly the African American Collaborative Obesity Research Network. Prior to the Council, Dr. Affuso was a tenured Associate Professor in the Department of Epidemiology at the University of Alabama at Birmingham. She is also a Senior Research Scientist with the Gramercy Research Group. Dr. Affuso previously served as co-Director of the Investigator Development Core for the UAB Obesity Health Disparities Research Center. In addition to having served as an advisor for various organizations, Dr. Affuso is the proud recipient of research funding from a variety of funders including the National Institutes of Health and the American Heart Association. She has been featured on globally recognized platforms such as TED, Disney+, and PBS. Outside of academic engagement, you can find Dr. Affuso serving as an ambassador for *Ultrarunning Magazine* and Altrarunning, supporting girls through her role with the Grassroots Community Foundation, and maintaining her four-year-plus streak of running at least 1 mile every day. She obtained her PhD in Nutrition Epidemiology from the University of North Carolina at Chapel Hill. She also completed a postdoctoral fellowship in the Department of Exercise and Sport Sciences at the University of Miami.

Shawn Arango Ricks, PhD, M.Ed., Chair, Department of Leadership and Educational Studies, Associate Professor, Social & Philosophical Foundations of Education, Reich College of Education, Appalachian State University

Dr. Shawn Arango Ricks combines her lived experiences with more than 20 years of research and teaching. Dr. Ricks has a passion for helping individuals and organizations thrive. She is passionate about creating spaces where individuals can lead "well"—meaning they maintain their health and wellness within organizational cultures. Her personal experience with burnout, as well as her work as a therapist, fuel her passion to help people learn strategies and tools to navigate life and work. For organizations, Dr. Ricks is committed to helping them create spaces where employees can thrive.

Dr. Ricks helps women debunk the myth of the superwoman and grind culture, and uses her skills as a coach, teacher, and trainer to guide others to creating their most joy-filled lives. She has created two highly successful empowerment programs, Sojourn to Self and No Mask, No Cape, and is the author of two books: *Write Your Own Story: A Handbook* and *Psychological Tight Spaces: One Black Feminist Scholars' Journey Into Academia*. Dr. Ricks was formerly the Assistant Vice President for Equity, Diversity and Inclusion and an Associate Professor of Race and Ethnicity Studies at Salem Academy and College in Winston-Salem, NC. At Salem she worked with faculty, staff, and students around issues of equity, diversity and inclusion at both individual and institution levels. Prior to her appointment at Salem, Dr. Ricks was an associate professor of counseling and human services at Old Dominion University. Dr. Ricks has experience working with diverse student populations, and has worked in the community college system, an HBCU, large public and small private settings. She received her PhD from the University of North Carolina at Greensboro in Educational Leadership and Cultural Foundations, and a Masters in Counselor Education from the Pennsylvania State University, University Park. Dr. Ricks is also a Licensed Clinical Mental Health Counselor, and a Licensed Clinical Addictions Specialist. She is the current president of the North Carolina Foundation for Alcohol and Drug Studies, and a past president of the Southern Organization for Human Services. Dr. Ricks serves as an editor for the *Journal of Human Services*, and is a reviewer for the *Urban Review* and the *Journal of Curriculum Theorizing*. Her research interests include the psychosocial well-being of Black women, epistemic injustice, and holistic approaches to gendered racism and trauma for Black women and girls.

Y. Falami Devoe, PhD, MA, Antioch University

Dr. Y. "Falami" Devoe is a Womanist, Participatory Action Research Scholar-Activist, PhotoArtist, and poet with interdisciplinary interests at the intersections of race, class, gender, identity, sexuality, ethnography, and pedagogy. Dr. Falami's work documents Black women's experiences of resilience, resistance, agency, and affirmation. She is passionate about the voices of Black women and how critical these voices are in creating new narratives and sustainable practices of healing, liberation, and well-being. She creates and curates spaces for Black women to express themselves authentically and to help make meaning of their lived experiences of their bodies. As an activist, scholar, practitioner, Dr. Falami integrates mindfulness, art, poetry, storytelling, and photography in her courses and presentations. Dr. Falami's work brings attention to the Photovoice methodology as an affirming and culturally relevant methodological approach that fosters a legacy of stories and experiences via pictures and words for marginalized communities. She received her PhD from the Graduate School of Leadership and Change from Antioch University and her MA in Leadership and Change and her MA in Educational Leadership from Antioch University and a BA from Hampton University. She is a Certified Holistic Health Coach and a proud member of Delta Sigma Theta Sorority, Inc.

Danielle Dickens, PhD, MS, Spelman College

Danielle Dickens, PhD, joined the department of psychology as an assistant professor in 2015. She received her bachelor's degree in psychology from Spelman College, and her master's and doctorate degrees in applied social and health psychology from Colorado State University. Dr. Dickens uses an interdisciplinary approach and pulls together her knowledge and experience as an instructor and mentor around issues of race/ethnicity, gender, age, and class in higher education and the workplace. As a Black feminist social psychologist, her research focuses on the identity development and identity formation of Black women and how they navigate the world. She utilizes qualitative and quantitative methodologies to examine the intersection of multiple identities, specifically race, gender, age, and class identities, with an emphasis on Black women, work, higher education, and STEM.

Dr. Dickens is most interested in examining how members of underrepresented groups (e.g., Black women) experience discrimination, the utilization of identity shifting as a coping strategy, and the benefits and costs of identity shifting on Black women's physical and mental health. In her second line of research, she examines the social-psychological determinants of academic and career development of Black women.

LeConté J. Dill, Michigan State University, Department of African American and African Studies

Dr. LeConté J. Dill is a community-accountable educator, scholar, and artist born and raised in South Central Los Angeles. Currently, she is an Associate Professor in the Department of African American and African Studies at Michigan State University. She is also a Certified Mindfulness Instructor. Dr. Dill's scholarship is critically informed by years of working in partnership with youth and community organizers, health educators, and policy advocates at community-based organizations and public health departments across the

United States. In her art, scholarship, and activism, she listens to and shows up for urban Black girls and works to rigorously document their experiences of safety, resilience, resistance, and wellness.

Sara Flowers, DrPH, Vice President, Education & Training, Planned Parenthood Federation of America

Dr. Sara C. Flowers is the Vice President of Education & Training at Planned Parenthood Federation of America. Planned Parenthood is the nation's largest provider of sex education, providing expert information, resources, and guidance to parents, caregivers, and young people, both online and in communities across the country. Dr. Flowers's passion for sex education began as a high school student, when she led the Annual AIDS Awareness Day for her peers at Spring Valley Senior High School in the late 1990s. Since then, she has written, implemented, and evaluated sex education programs and curricula for Boys and Girls Clubs of Greater Washington, the George Washington University Student Health Service, the Association of Reproductive Health Professionals, and Cornell University Cooperative Extension—New York City. Prior to joining PPFA, Dr. Flowers was Director of Youth Initiatives for Love Heals Center for Youth & Families at GMHC. In this role, she expanded existing and launched new programs, as well as oversaw sex education and leadership program curriculum development and revision. She also coordinated quantitative and qualitative program evaluation and reporting; cultivated and maintained community partnerships; and hired, trained, and managed staff and a freelance health education team. Concurrently, Dr. Flowers was an adjunct assistant professor for York College, CUNY while serving as a Post-Doctoral Research Fellow for the college's Collaborative Research Group on Health Policy & Promotion + the Urban-Health Lab.

Dr. Flowers previously served as a member of the Boards of Directors of both the New York Abortion Access Fund (NYAAF) and SIECUS: Sex Ed for Social Change. She is a member of Women of Color Sexual Health Network (WOCSHN), a trainer on emotional intelligence with Equilibrium Dynamics in San Francisco, and a published author. Her most recent publications are "Sisterhood Unexpected: 'I Met My Best Friend in LEAP!' and Other Narratives by LEAP for Girls Alumnae New York City, 2006–2016" (2022), and "Enacting Our Multidimensional Power: Black Women Sex Educators Demonstrate the Value of an Intersectional Sexuality Education Framework" (2018). Dr. Flowers holds a Doctorate in Public Health from The Graduate School and University Center, CUNY, as well as a BA in Psychology and a Master of Public Health degree, both from the George Washington University.

Juliette Marion Garofolo, BS, The George Washington University

Juliette Marion Garofolo has a Bachelor of Science from The George Washington University where she graduated Summa Cum Laude majoring in Public Health and Women, Gender, and Sexuality Studies. Her interests lie at the intersection of community health and sexual health, specifically within marginalized communities. Juliette currently works as a paralegal in immigration law at The Law Office of Craig Relles. She seeks to attend law school to merge her passions for community, public health, and policy to make the world a more equitable place.

Linda Goler Blount, MPH, President & CEO (Alias: The Black Magic Woman)

Linda Goler Blount joined the Black Women's Health Imperative as the president and chief executive officer in February 2014. As president and CEO, Linda oversees the strategic direction for the Imperative and is responsible for moving the organization forward in its mission to achieve health equity, as well as reproductive justice for Black women.

Before joining the Imperative, Linda served as the vice president of programmatic impact for the United Way of Greater Atlanta, where she led the effort to eliminate inequalities in health, income, education, and housing through place- and population-based work. Prior to that position, Linda was the first-ever national vice president of health disparities at the American Cancer Society. There, she was responsible for providing strategic vision and leadership to the Society and its 12 geographic divisions to reduce cancer incidence and mortality among underserved populations and to develop a nationwide health equity policy.

With more than 25 years of experience in the public, for-profit and non-profit sectors, Linda has a distinguished career that includes successful tenures at The Coca-Cola Company, leading strategic business initiatives, and the U.S. Centers for Disease Control and Prevention, as an expert scientist. She also has extensive international health expertise and has served as a consultant to government ministries in Germany, South Africa, Zimbabwe, Malawi, Jamaica, and Trinidad and Tobago, where she lived for four years. Linda is a sought-after speaker and a member of the American Public Health Association and the National Association of Health Services Executives. She serves on the Community Health Charities Board, the University of Michigan School of Public Health Summer Enrichment Program Board and is past chair of the University of Michigan School of Public Health Alumni Board of Governors. She previously served on the Emory University Center for Ethics Advisory Board, and the Morehouse School of Medicine Public Health Program Advisory Committee. A Michigan native, Linda holds a Master of Public Health degree in Epidemiology from the University of Michigan and a Bachelor of Science in Computer Engineering/Operations Research from Eastern Michigan University.

Carlysha Isaac, MPhil

Carlysha Isaac currently works at the U.S Department of State. She has an MPhil in International Peace Studies at Trinity College Dublin and a BA in Psychology at Towson University. She has previously written about prioritizing mental health as a Black American woman living abroad for Ezi Health.

Dr. Maryam M. Jernigan-Noesi, Med, PhD, Founder, CEO, Jernigan & Associates Psychology and Educational Consulting LLC

Dr. Jernigan-Noesi is a licensed psychologist, clinical researcher, former professor, and consultant with over two decades of experience in mental health. She has extensive training and work experiences in child psychology, women's health, and specialized training in youth, adult, and family interventions. She frequently serves as a consultant nationally for school districts, colleges, and universities to offer guidance on promoting equity and reducing experiences of marginalization and discrimination.

Dr. Jernigan-Noesi completed advanced clinical training at The Center for Multicultural Training in Psychology at Boston Medical Center and Boston University School of Medicine. She also completed post-doctoral fellowships at Harvard Medical School and Yale University School of Medicine. She is the Director of the Intersections Research Lab, where she focuses on understanding the impact of gendered racism and race-related stress and trauma on mental and physical health outcomes across the lifespan. As a former professor, Dr. Maryam taught undergraduate, graduate, and professional students across the health disciplines for over 15 years. Her expertise has led to numerous elected appointments and advising roles. She serves as an advisor for the Sesame Street racial justice initiative. She is a member of the Advisory Board for Camp HOPE America—the leading year-round camping and mentoring program in the United States for children and teens impacted by domestic violence. Dr. Jernigan-Noesi was appointed to the Board of Directors for the Boyce L. Ansley School, a tuition-free private school for children and families who have experienced homelessness.

Breya Johnson, MS, writer, researcher, and Black feminist cultural worker

Breya M. Johnson is a writer, researcher, and Black feminist cultural worker. She runs the Instagram blog @blackreadingtoheal. Her work looks at reproductive justice, care ethics, Black feminisms, and Black women's inner workings.

Toni Junious, MPH, Milken Institute School of Public Health, George Washington University, Washington, DC and Black Women's Health Imperative, Washington, DC

Toni Lynn Junious, MPH, is a public health and holistic wellness practitioner passionate about improving health and health equity in her community. She has worked in women's wellness, disease prevention, community outreach, and qualitative and quantitative community-based research to increase access to resources to help individuals reach optimal health and well-being. Toni graduated from University of California, Irvine with a Bachelor of Arts in Public Health and Global Cultures, and a minor in Medical Anthropology. She received her Masters of Public Health (MPH) in Global Health Epidemiology at the George Washington University, Milken Institute School of Public Health. Toni is the co-founder of Soultry Sisters, an arts and wellness collective that empowers women of color to cultivate vibrant lives through soulcare, sustainability, and collective healing. Learn more about her work at SoultrySisters.com. Toni is also a 200 HR-certified yoga teacher, community herbalist, and full-spectrum doula. Through a holistic approach, she blends health equity, sexual and reproductive justice, and empowerment to address the root causes of disease and promote wellness as liberation.

Shiriki K. Kumanyika, PhD, MPH, MS, Founding Chair, Council on Black Hair and Research Professor, Community Health and Prevention, Drexel University Dornsife School of Public Health

Dr. Shiriki Kumanyika is Emeritus Professor of epidemiology in the Department of Biostatistics and Epidemiology at the University of Pennsylvania Perelman School of Medicine. She has an interdisciplinary background and holds advanced degrees in social work, nutrition, and public health. During her tenure on the Penn Medicine faculty, Dr. Kumanyika also served as the Associate Dean for Health Promotion and Disease Prevention, held a secondary appointment as Professor of Epidemiology in the Department of Pediatrics (Division of Gastroenterology, Nutrition Section), and was affiliated with numerous Penn institutes and centers. She was the Founding Director of Penn's interdisciplinary, multi-school Master of Public Health program. Dr. Kumanyika's research focuses on identifying effective strategies to reduce nutrition-related chronic disease risks, with a particular focus on achieving health equity for Black Americans. Dr. Kumanyika founded (in 2002) and led the African American Collaborative Obesity Research Network (AACORN), a national network, until 2018 when AACORN took on a broader mission and rebranded as the Council on Black Health (www.councilbh.org). She was Vice-Chair of the HHS Secretary's Advisory Committee on Healthy People 2020 objectives, was president of the American Public Health Association, is a member of the

National Academy of Medicine (NAM), and current chair of the NAM Food and Nutrition Board. Dr. Kumanyika is also a nutrition advisor to the World Health Organization and the World Cancer Research Fund, and Chair of the Expert Group for the Access to Nutrition Initiative.

Martha Kakooza, Morgan State University

Martha Kakooza grew up in Kampala, Uganda. She moved to Baltimore in 2012 and in the years that followed her move, she gained a growing interest in transnationalism. Currently, she is learning to become a scholar-practitioner whose work (both in scholarship and practice) is focused on the intersection of gender, immigration, and Black livelihood. Her practice and programming are rooted in Africana womanism with the hopes of documenting lived and felt experiences through storying. You can always find Martha sipping on a hot cup of tea (even during the summer) or listening to a podcast.

Afiya Mbilishaka, PhD, Psychologist, Hairstylist, Founder/CEO, Pschohairapy

Being in love with hair her whole life, Dr. Afiya grew up as her family's hairstylist, graduating from lawn chairs at cookouts to eventually holding space in her college dorm room for a mini-salon. Her trait of being a skillful active listener translated smoothly to the field of psychology, earning her degrees from the University of Pennsylvania and Howard University. At the age of 26, Dr. Afiya earned a PhD in Clinical Psychology and was a full-time therapist at Columbia University and then she was a professor at the University of the District of Columbia. Dr. Afiya is a natural hairstylist and partners with N Natural Hair Studio in Silver Spring, Maryland where she loves creating art with locs, twists, and afros.

Chinyere Okafor, The Graduate Center, CUNY

Chinyere Okafor (she/dey/they) is a writer, healing arts practitioner, facilitator, and a PhD candidate at The Graduate Center, CUNY in the Critical Social/Personality and Environmental Psychology program. Her research interests are on race and space, Black marginalized genders' narratives in higher education, and alternative healing modalities for Black mental health. Chinyere has contributed to *Meridians: feminism, race, transnationalism* and *Stories Changing Lives: Narratives and Paths Toward Social Change*. They are also a co-founder of Tar Beach, an interior design studio that uses transnational Black feminism to bridge Black folks' relationships with themselves, their sacred spaces, healing arts, and learning.

Madelyn Stalter, under/graduate public health student, The George Washington University

Madelyn Stalter, BS/MPH, is student at the George Washington University studying Community-Oriented Primary Care.

Tambra Raye Stevenson, MPH, MA, Founder, WANDA

Tambra Raye Stevenson, MPH, MA, founded WANDA: Women Advancing Nutrition, Dietetics, and Agriculture with a mission to empower Black women and girls who lead healthier communities through sustainable food systems in Africa and the diaspora. She is a PhD candidate at the American University School of Communication, delving into the intricate intersection of media, technology, and health. She is a communication researcher in the NSF-funded Wasted Food Research Network, led by American University. Supporting policy-makers and practitioners, her food and health communication research agenda centers on Black women and addresses structural communication inequalities within under-resourced communities. Tambra's scholarly journey began with bench lab, clinical nutrition, and community-based nutrition research, collaborating with esteemed researchers such as Dr. Shiriki Kumanyika, Dr. Karen Peterson, and Dr. Stephen Abrams. Tambra's influence extends beyond academia, as she is the principal author of the Black Health Bill of Rights, adopted by the Council on Black Health, a network of academic researchers and community partners.

She earned her Bachelor's degree in Human Nutrition with a Spanish minor from Oklahoma State University, where she also studied community health in the Dominican Republic as a recipient of the prestigious David L. Boren National Security Scholarship. She earned her MPH in Health Communication from Tufts University School of Medicine and pursued MBA coursework in entrepreneurship and healthcare marketing at Boston University Graduate School of Management. Tambra's public service career began in roles focused on the social determinants of health, such as the Secretary's office of the U.S. Department of Health and Human Services, the U.S. Department of Commerce's Minority Business Development Agency, the Executive Office of the D.C. Mayor on Women's Policy and Initiatives, D.C. Victim Services, and at the University of the District of Columbia's Center for Nutrition, Diet, and Health. Additionally, Tambra holds a design patent pending and authored WANDA's children's bilingual book series. With her extensive expertise and accomplishments, Tambra is a highly sought-after speaker, facilitator, and consultant locally and globally. She has delivered impactful presentations at renowned events and institutions, including the Food Tank Summit, the World Bank/IMF Annual Meetings, United Nations Commission on the Status of Women NGO Forum, the U.S. Botanic Garden, the Children's National Medical Center, and various esteemed universities and organizations across Europe, Africa, and the Americas.

Maranda Ward, EdD, MPH, Assistant Professor and Director of Equity, Department of Clinical Research and Leadership, GW School of Medicine and Health Sciences

Executive Director, Promising Futures

Dr. Maranda C. Ward is an Assistant Professor and Director of Equity in the Department of Clinical Research and Leadership in the GW School of Medicine and Health Sciences. Dr. Ward is an expert in advancing anti-racism efforts within health professions education and in designing curricula to enable students and faculty to competently promote health and racial equity in practice. Her research focuses on educational interventions as well as stakeholder-engaged community-focused studies on HIV, Black women's health, and youth identity. Her earliest publication was a direct result of a research fellowship where she conducted a literature search and secondary analysis of a data set on covariates of adolescent intimate partner violence of the SAFE DATES Program (Ward & McMahon, 2006). Her next set of publications stem from experience designing and evaluating service-learning, sexual health, and youth development programs and curriculum for adolescents (and young adults) in school and out of school contexts (Ward & Bullock, 2008; Ward, 2015; Ward, 2017; Ward, 2020). More recently, she served as the first and senior author of work published in Medical Education (Ward & Ganjoo, 2022) and MedEdPortal (Falusi et al., 2023), respectively, on advancing community-based research to advance social justice and faculty development for racial/health equity. In addition to educational research, a primary area of focus of her scholarship is advancing anti-racism and intersectionality research, as evidenced in a research handbook on developing competencies for pre-health students (Ward et al., 2022) and a chapter in an APHA press textbook on Black women's reproductive and sexual health (Ward, et. al., 2023). As a member of the DC Center for AIDS Research (DC CFAR), she is the principal investigator of Two in One: HIV and COVID Screening & Testing Model that allows her to lead national research-based educational intervention for primary care practitioners to routinize screening and testing for HIV, PrEP, and the COVID-19 vaccine.

Melicia C. Whitt-Glover, PhD, President and CEO, Gramercy Research Group, and Executive Director, Council on Black Health, Inc.

Dr. Melicia Whitt-Glover is President and CEO of Gramercy Research Group in Winston Salem, NC. Gramercy Research Group's mission is to positively impact and improve the lives of individuals and communities by addressing health and related issues. She is also Executive Director for the Council on Black Health, Inc. The Council's mission is to develop and promote solutions that achieve health in Black communities. For over 20 years, Dr. Whitt-Glover has been engaged in research and evaluation projects designed to identify effective strategies to promote adherence to national recommendations for physical activity, diet, and healthy weight gain to address disparities in chronic disease morbidity and mortality. Her research has been funded by the National Institutes of Health, the Patient Centered Outcomes Research Institute, national and local foundations, and local government organizations. She was a member of the 2018 Physical Activity Guidelines Advisory Committee, which was a group of the country's most accomplished physical activity and health experts who will play a critical role in a comprehensive process, culminating with the publication of the second edition of the *Physical Activity Guidelines* for Americans. Dr. Whitt-Glover received her BA (Exercise Physiology, 1993) and MA (Exercise Physiology, 1996) from the University of North Carolina at Chapel Hill. She received her PhD (Epidemiology, 1999) from the University of South Carolina. Dr. Whitt-Glover completed a postdoctoral fellowship at the University of Pennsylvania School of Medicine (2000–2002).

Danielle Whyte, The George Washington University

Danielle Whyte, The George Washington University. Author of scholarly works 'Black Girl Magic': A Radiant Response to Oppression and The Harsh and Deadly Effects of the 'Strong, Independent Black Woman Trope'.

www.ingramcontent.com/pod-product-compliance
Lightning Source LLC
Chambersburg PA
CBHW051256200926
51612CB00002B/63
9781666911749